IMMUNOINFORMATICS OF CANCERS

IMMUNOINFORMATICS OF CANCERS

PRACTICAL MACHINE LEARNING APPROACHES USING R

NIMA REZAEI

Research Center for Immunodeficiencies, Tehran University of Medical Sciences, Tehran, Iran

PARNIAN JABBARI

Network of Immunity in Infection, Malignancy and Autoimmunity (NIIMA), Universal Scientific Education and Research Network (USERN), Tehran, Iran

ELSEVIER

ACADEMIC PRESS

An imprint of Elsevier

Academic Press is an imprint of Elsevier
125 London Wall, London EC2Y 5AS, United Kingdom
525 B Street, Suite 1650, San Diego, CA 92101, United States
50 Hampshire Street, 5th Floor, Cambridge, MA 02139, United States
The Boulevard, Langford Lane, Kidlington, Oxford OX5 1GB, United Kingdom

ISBN: 978-0-12-822400-7

For Information on all Academic Press publications
visit our website at https://www.elsevier.com/books-and-journals

Publisher: Andre G. Wolff
Acquisitions Editor: Glyn Jones
Editorial Project Manager: Ivy Dawn Torre
Production Project Manager: Punithavathy Govindaradjane
Cover Designer: Mark Rogers

Typeset by MPS Limited, Chennai, India

Dedication

To all those fighting cancer, one way or another.

Contents

Section II

Basics of R programming

Section III

ML algorithms and their applications

Preface

Machine learning (ML) and artificial intelligence (AI) have revolutionized every field over the past decades, with life sciences being no exception. High-throughput experimentsproduce massive volumes of data that are hard to deal with using conventional statistical methods. In addition, these statistical methods cannot encompass all aspects of such data and are incapable of discovering new relationships among different data components.

In the beginning, AI- and ML-powered algorithms were used only by professionals in related fields, such as computer sciences. With interdisciplinary research becoming more and more common, the use of AI and ML is fast gaining importance in research in every scientific field to the extent that at least basic knowledge of these algorithms is deemed necessary for all researchers, and researchers from various fields are getting more and more familiar with applications and potentials of these algorithmsHowever, learning the principles of these algorithms can be challenging for researchers from different backgrounds.

This book is designed to introduce principles of ML in the context of cancer immunology. Authors considered the diverse audience the book can attract, especially researchers from biological and computational fields who wish to conduct interdisciplinary research involving biology and computer sciences, what is commonly known as bioinformatics. In this book, ML algorithms are implemented in the R environment, since R is one of the most common platforms of programming in bioinformatics. The main difference of this book from other similar titles is in the way it approaches complicated concepts, such as programming, or ML algorithms, which can prove to be encouraging to researchers. These concepts are overviewed in a simple, yet practical manner, which allows a better understanding of the concepts for all readers. The computational aspects of most algorithms have been discussed in an easy-to-follow manner for interested readers. Another key feature of this book is introduction to several ML algorithms available today and then comparing outcomes from different algorithms to help readers better understand the principles and applications of these ML algorithms. Unlike other books on ML that include examples with perfect data sets that result in perfect models without any challenges, authors have tried to include challenges that can be frustrating for the readers if faced independently.

The book is divided in three broad sections. The first section is dedicated to introducing biological aspects, the second section covers basics of R programming, and the third section deals with most common ML algorithms and their applications in cancer bioinformatics. Chapter 1 discusses roles of the immune system, and how it can fight cancers. This chapter can be of special interest to readers from life sciences. Chapter 2 introduces bioinformatics as an interdisciplinary field and overviews some of the commonly used tools in bioinformatics. Chapter 3 introduces some of the useful online tools and databases used in cancer immunoinformatics. Chapter 4 overviews principles of R programming that are relevant to ML approaches discussed in this book. Chapter 5 introduces ML and its basic concepts, which lay the foundation for future chapters. Chapter 6 is dedicated to the Naive Bayes classification, and Chapter 7 introduces two of the most commonly used regression and classification algorithms: linear and logistic regression. Chapter 8 deals with discriminant-based classifiers, focusing on linear and quadratic discriminant analyses. Chapters 9–12 provide examples of applying support vector machine, decision trees, random forests, and K-nearest neighbors for classification and regression problems. Chapter 13 briefly introduces neural networks, focusing on supervised learning applications while providing examples for unsupervised applications. Chapter 14 applies the algorithms discussed throughout the book on real-world data, providing several examples for ML in bioinformatics.

Evidently, this book cannot be considered as a book to master ML, which is beyond its scope; however, it can be a good starting point and a comprehensive guide for researchers who wish to include ML in their research. Finally, authors appreciate any valuable suggestions or criticisms leading to more enhanced future editions of this title.

Nima Rezaei
Parnian Jabbari

SECTION I

Biological aspects

CHAPTER

1

Introduction to cancer immunology

An introduction to the immune system

Any living organism is armed against its surrounding and intrinsic pathogenic factors by several means, including its immune system. The complexity of the immune system varies from one organism to another depending on its evolution [1]. We can broadly divide the immune system into innate or adaptive (acquired) immunity [2]. The innate immune system can be further divided into physical and chemical arms. Physical barriers of the immune system such as the skin and the cilia prevent the pathogens from entering the body. The chemical arm, however, is usually more complicated and has the ability to partly eliminate pathogens in a nonspecific manner through means such as low pH, phagocytosis, inflammation, etc. [2]. Innate immunity is the first line of protection in an organism; therefore, it has to be rapid in responding against pathogens. Due to this rapidness, no memory against a specific pathogen is created. Furthermore, innate immunity is not specific and exhibits the same behavior in facing different pathogens. Many cells serve in the innate immune system: phagocytes, neutrophils, basophils, mast cells, phagocytes, natural killer (NK) cells, eosinophils, and dendritic cells (DCs). These cells play various roles, from antigen presentation (DCs and macrophages) to cytokine production [3]. In addition to blood and tissue cells mentioned earlier, the innate immune system consists of blood proteins, such as cytokines, and components of the complement system that help in the elimination of pathogens. Even though the innate immune system is effective against many pathogens, there are

Immunoinformatics of Cancers
DOI: https://doi.org/10.1016/B978-0-12-822400-7.00008-7

numerous pathogens that can resist the responses of the innate immune system. That is why one of the most important roles of the innate immune system is the activation of the adaptive immune responses.

The adaptive immune system, which is found only in jawed vertebrates, unlike the innate immune system, exhibits specific immune responses. These immune responses are slower to commence and can be memorized, which can provide the organism with long-term immunity against a specific pathogen. The adaptive immune system can be divided into humoral and cell-mediated immunity [2].

Humoral immunity

There are various macromolecules that play roles in humoral immunity. These macromolecules that include antimicrobial peptides, antibodies, and proteins of the complement system are all found in body fluids, including plasma, interstitial fluid, and mucosa. Antibodies can be considered the most important components of humoral immunity, which are produced by B lymphocytes (B cells) [4]. B cells are produced and matured in the bone marrow. During their maturation in bone marrow, B cells go through random gene rearrangements that result in the production of B cells with millions of antigenic specificities [2]. Antibodies that are produced by a specific type of B cells called plasma cells are specific to each antigen. An antigen is any molecule that can bind to antibodies. Once the binding of an antigen to an antibody leads to an immune response, the antigen also becomes an immunogen. However, these two terms are usually used interchangeably. Antigens have specific parts that can be recognized by the immune system (antibodies or lymphocyte receptors); these parts are called determinants or epitopes [2]. Once an epitope is recognized by an antibody, it either eliminates the pathogen/toxin or stimulates mechanisms that lead to its elimination, and in the case of an antibody on the surface of B cells (B-cell receptor, BCR), it activates the B cells and leads to clonal expansion, which is increased proliferation of B cells with that specific BCR. Furthermore, memory B cells are produced after the recognition of a specific antigen and produce antibodies with higher affinity (stronger immune response) to that antigen [5].

An individual is armed with millions of different antibodies with a unique antigen-binding specificity. These antibodies can be grouped into five antibody classes as IgA, IgD, IgE, IgG, and IgM. These antibodies are structurally slightly different; however, they have some structural characteristics in common: all antibodies have asymmetric structure and consist of two identical light chains and two identical heavy chains. Each antibody has an antigen-binding fragment (Fab) and a crystallizing fragment consisting of CH_2 and CH_3 domains (Fc). The coding genes for the antigen-binding region of antibodies undergo somatic hypermutation during the proliferation of B cells, and this leads to the expansion of the B-cell repertoire. Fig. 1.1 delineates the principal structure of antibodies.

Cell-mediated immunity

T lymphocytes (T cells) are responsible for the elimination of intracellular pathogens by either destruction of the pathogens or killing of the host cells in which the pathogens reside [2]. They exercise these functions either directly or by recruitment of other white blood cells (leukocytes) such as phagocytes and B cells. Unlike B cells, which can

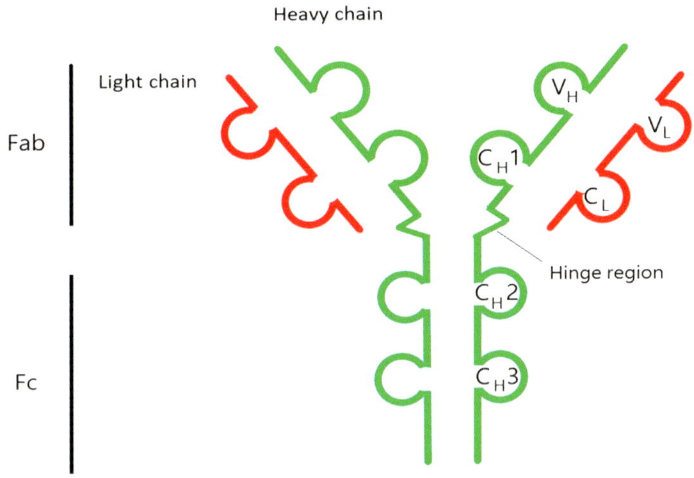

FIGURE 1.1 Antibody structure: Each antibody has two identical light chains and two identical heavy chains. The variable regions of the heavy chain and the light chain, along with the constant region of the light chain and the first constant region of the heavy chain (CH1), compose the antibody-binding fragment (Fab). The antigen-binding site is part of Fab and consists of variable regions of the heavy and the light chains. The second and third (and in the case of membrane-bound antibodies, the fourth) constant regions of heavy chains compose the crystallizable fragment (Fc) that exert the effector mechanism of the antibody. The hinge grants flexibility to the antibody by permitting independent movement in this region. Even though the humoral immunity is effective against many pathogens, for those pathogens that are intracellular, like viral or certain bacterial infections, the cell-mediated (cellular) adaptive immunity is in charge of the elimination of the pathogens or cells infected with that pathogen.

recognize antigens irrespective of their chemical and physical features or where they may be presented, T cells can only recognize antigens presented on the surface of cells. Even though T cells have a large antigenic repertoire, there are limited numbers of each T cell-specific to an antigen. Therefore, there is a need for a system to capture antigens and deliver them to lymphoid organs in which T cells can encounter the antigens [2]. Antigen-presenting cells (APCs) are cells that present antigens to T cells. Despite the fact that all nucleated cells can present antigens to some T cells in different situations, the term APC does not apply to all of these cells.

There are various types of T cells based on the cluster-of-differentiation (CD) markers expressed on the surface of T cells. Two of the most important T cells based on their CD expression are CD4 + and CD8 + T cells, which represent helper T cells (Th cells) and cytotoxic T lymphocytes (CTLs), respectively [2]. In order for T cells to recognize antigens, which in the case of T cells are mostly peptides, they must be bound to major histocompatibility complex (MHC) molecules. CD4 + T cells recognize antigens that are bound to class I MHC molecules, and CD8 + T cells recognize those bound to class II MHC molecules. MHC-antigen binding is an important topic in immunology, which will be further discussed under the "Antigen–MHC binding" section in this chapter.

The most important APCs presenting antigens to CD4 + T cells are DCs [6]. DCs are present in virtually all tissues, and they express receptors on their surface that bind to microbes, ingest the microbes, and present the processed antigens of the microbe bound to MHC-I molecules on their surface. Once DCs recognize microbial antigens, they migrate to lymphoid organs where they chemically attract T cells [2]. Exposure of T cells to protein antigens presented by DCs leads to the activation of T cells, which can in turn further enhance innate immunity and B cell response.

Antigen–major histocompatibility complex binding

One of the most important topics in immunology and a challenge for bioinformaticians is the presentation of antigens by MHC molecules [7]. In humans, MHC molecules are called human leukocyte antigens (HLAs). MHC loci include more than 200 genes that are classified mainly into two types of highly polymorphic MHC genes of classes I and II, which encode the class I and II MHC molecules, respectively [8]. In some references, some genes of this group are categorized as class III genes, which encode molecules that serve the immune system in a nonpeptide presentation fashion. MHC genes are highly polymorphic, which means the gene has many forms (alleles of that gene) present across individuals.

This polymorphism leads to various alleles that encode more than 5000 proteins. This, combined with other factors, such as the fact that MHC genes are expressed codominantly and undergo high rates of crossover (exchange of homologous genetic material between a pair of chromosomes) during meiosis, is the basis for recognizing many pathogenic antigens by the immune system [8]. In humans, the MHC class I genes have three main subcategories: HLA-A, HLA-B, and HLA-C; however, there have been more subcategories identified that belong to the class I MHC genes [8]. Class II MHC genes contain six main HLA subcategories: HLA-DPA1, HLA-DPB1, HLA-DQA1, HLA-DQB1, HLA-DRA, and HLA-DRB1. These genes have various alleles, some of which are associated with immune-related diseases [9].

Class I MHC molecules are present on the surface of all nucleated cells, while class II MHC molecules are expressed on DCs, B lymphocytes, macrophages, as well as a few other cell types, and they present antigens to CD4 + T cells [8]. This pattern of expression of MHC molecules allows the immune system to recognize viral infections and malignant antigens in any cell by calling immune response from CD8 + T cells. Even though there are minor structural differences between the two classes of MHC molecules, both classes consist of a peptide-binding cleft, a transmembrane region, and an intracellular domain [8]. The peptide-binding cleft of MHC molecules is formed by the folding of the amino acids. As mentioned earlier, the MHC genes are highly polymorphic, so is the amino acid sequence of their products, which form the peptide-binding cleft. This allows MHC molecules to present many different peptides to T cells [8]. Despite the fact that each MHC molecule can bind to many different peptides based on their amino acid sequence, T cells can only recognize one specific peptide among the peptides MHC molecules present. Therefore, in order for T cells to recognize an antigen, all three components of including MHC, peptide's specific sequence, and T-cell receptor must be matching in order for T cells to exhibit immune response [10]. Fig. 1.2 illustrates a peptide presentation by MHC molecules of classes I and II.

X-ray crystallography has provided a large body of information regarding MHC–peptide complexes [10]. MHC I molecule can only present peptide fragments of 8–11 amino acid length. On the other hand, the peptide-binding cleft of MHC class II molecule can bind to peptides of 10–30 residues or longer. Furthermore, some MHC molecules have pockets with predilections for certain amino acids at certain sites of the sequence. Some amino acids in the binding peptide are anchor residues as they have side chains that bind to complementary structures on the MHC molecule. Such characteristics in the biding of MHC and peptide allow for the generation of algorithms to predict MHC–peptide binding [11].

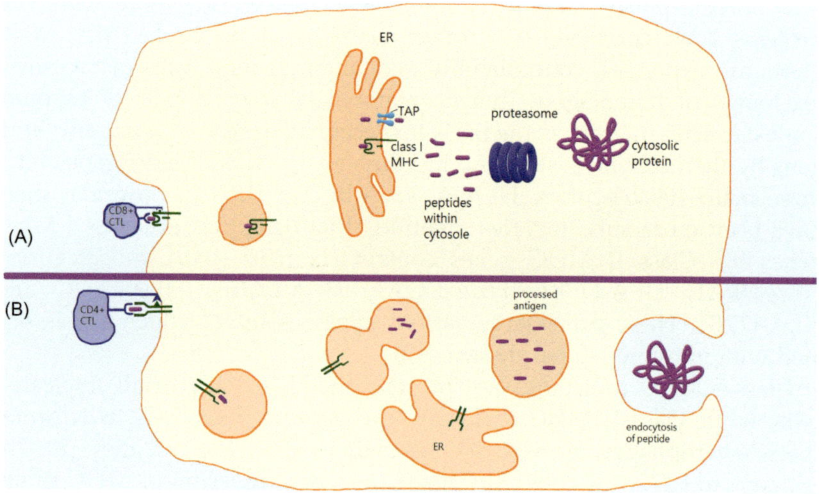

FIGURE 1.2 Major histocompatibility complex (MHC)–antigen binding. (A) In the class I MHC pathway, peptides are processed by the proteasome within the cytosol and are transported into the endoplasmic reticulum (ER) through a transporter associated with antigen processing (TAP). There, processed peptides bind MHC I molecules and are then presented on the surface of the antigen-presenting cells (APC). (B) In the class II MHC pathway, peptides are endocytosed and processed in the vesicles. The processed antigens are then presented by MHC II molecules on the surface of the cell.

Self-tolerance

Antigens present in an organism's own cells are known as self-antigens. These antigens, like foreign antigens, are presented to T cells by MHC molecules. However, T cells that recognize self-antigens are eliminated and do not exert an immunologic response against these antigens [12]. This discrimination against self-antigens is known as self-tolerance. Self-tolerance can occur at two levels: one at the level of central (generative) lymphoid organs (i.e., bone marrow and thymus) and the other at the level of peripheral lymphoid organs, such as spleen and lymph nodes. Many mechanisms induce self-tolerance. Some self-antigens are hidden from the immune system, thus not inducing immune responses. On the other hand, regulatory T cells (Treg) can suppress lymphocytes reactive to self-antigens. Those T cells that recognize self-antigens are eliminated either through apoptosis or through anergy or functional unresponsiveness of the immune system.

Even though immune cells are screened at many levels to minimize the immune response toward self-antigens, some immune cells that are responsive to self-antigens can evade these screening mechanisms and cause autoimmune diseases [13].

Immunology of cancers

Many observations support that the immune system responds to malignancies. Histopathologic studies of the tumors show infiltration of the immune cells such as NK cells and macrophages in the tumor, which is associated with a better outcome [14]. As the immune system can discriminate self-antigens from non-self-antigens, it also can detect the changes that occur in self-antigens, which is the case for malignancies. Malignant cells are immunogens as they can provoke immune responses; however, the extent to which they activate the immune system depends on a variety of factors [15]. One of these factors is the immunocompetency of the host, as immunocompromised individuals have a greater risk of developing cancer. Another factor is the immunogenicity of the tumor antigens. Tumors can express antigens that are unique to malignant cells, which are termed tumor-specific antigens, or they can express antigens that can be found in normal cells as well, but their level of expression in malignant cells is different from that of normal cells, known as tumor-associated antigens (TAAs). Even though humoral immunity can help with the elimination of tumor cells either by activating the complement system or through cell-mediated cytotoxicity, the most important armor against malignant cells is the cellular immunity. Tumor antigens can be presented by MHC molecules on the cell surface, or they can be presented by DCs to T lymphocytes. CD8 + T cells play a major role in eliminating malignancies [16]. APCs, especially DCs, play important roles in presenting tumor antigens to CD8 + T cells and provide them with costimulatory signals that differentiate T cells from antitumor CTLs [17].

Many factors contribute to the recognition of tumor cells by antitumor CTLs. Cytokines, such as tumor necrosis factor and interferons, can promote the antitumor activity of CTLs by increasing the expression of MHC molecules on the surface of tumor cells, hence better presentation of antigens and stronger antitumor immune response [18]. However, despite the presence of effective mechanisms of the immune system to eliminate tumor cells, many tumors have developed strategies to evade the immune responses. One strategy is immunoediting: tumor cells can reduce the expression of antigens that do not favor tumor progression but rather call for immune response through high levels of immunogenicity [19]. In other words, tumors downregulate (i.e., reduce the expression of) genes that produce highly immunogenic antigens. Despite the efforts of cytokines to increase the expression of MHC molecules, tumors can downregulate the expression of these molecules, thus escaping immune recognition. On the other hand, tumors can grow independent of the growth factors, and they create a microenvironment that is favorable to their progression but hostile to the host immune cells [20]. Tumors can go further and suppress the immune system. They can produce immunosuppressive cytokines, such as tumor growth factor-beta (TGF-β) as well as free radicals, and disrupt the function of CTLs. Studies on immunologic aspects of cancers have drawn attention toward immunotherapy of cancers as one of the effective strategies to fight cancers.

Immunotherapy of cancers

Previous treatments of cancers were mostly confined to chemotherapy and radiotherapy. Despite being successful and being the mainstay of treatment in the case of many malignancies, these treatments are associated with serious adverse effects. Nonspecific inhibitory mechanisms of chemotherapeutic agents in eliminating cancer cells through interfering with cell proliferation cause tremendous damage to normal cells of the individual [21]. Understanding the pathways involved in the emergence and progression of cancers has enabled us to specifically target them. Immunotherapy is one of the promising approaches to the treatment of cancers [21]. Even though it does not entirely replace chemotherapy or radiotherapy in the case of many malignancies, it has changed the face of treatment in many cancers. Immunotherapy can enhance the host's immune responses to tumors through the recruitment of cytokines and their agonists, vaccines composed of killed malignant cells or their purified antigens, and enhancing TAA presentation by incubating DCs with tumor antigens [21]. Monoclonal antibodies (mAbs) revolutionized immunotherapy. They are antibodies that bind a certain antigen and can enhance antibody-mediated cellular cytotoxicity against tumor cells. Furthermore, mAbs can be used to deliver toxic agents directly to tumor cells. Another important application of mAbs is engineering chimeric antigen receptor T cells. By anchoring mAbs on T cells, they act as antigen receptors, which help T cells recognize TAAs in an MHC-independent manner. With the help of bioinformatics tools, T cells can also be engineered to detect more than one antigen at the same time and exert antitumor activity only when all the targeted antigens are detected. This can eliminate the unspecific toxicity of immunotherapy [21]. However, the role of bioinformatics in cancer therapy is beyond engineering potent anticancer T cells and it can improve the fight against cancers in several ways. In future chapters, we will focus on some uses of bioinformatics and computational biology in malignancies.

References

[1] J. Kaufman, Evolution and immunity, Immunology 130 (4) (2010) 459–462. Available from: https://doi.org/10.1111/j.1365-2567.2010.03294.x.
[2] D.D. Chaplin, Overview of the immune response, The Journal of Allergy and Clinical Immunology 125 (Suppl. 2) (2010) S3–S23. Available from: https://doi.org/10.1016/j.jaci.2009.12.980.
[3] S.E. Turvey, D.H. Broide, Innate immunity, The Journal of Allergy and Clinical Immunology 125 (2) (2010) S24–S32. Available from: https://doi.org/10.1016/j.jaci.2009.07.016.
[4] M.C. Carroll, Complement and humoral immunity, Vaccine 26 (Suppl. 8) (2008) I28–I33. Available from: https://doi.org/10.1016/j.vaccine.2008.11.022.
[5] W. Ratajczak, P. Niedźwiedzka-Rystwej, B. Tokarz-Deptuła, W. Deptuła, Immunological memory cells, Central European Journal of Immunology 43 (2) (2018) 194–203. Available from: https://doi.org/10.5114/ceji.2018.77390.
[6] M. Nakayama, Antigen presentation by MHC-dressed cells, Frontiers in Immunology 5 (2015) 672. Available from: https://doi.org/10.3389/fimmu.2014.00672. Published 2015 Jan 5.
[7] D. Gfeller, M. Bassani-Sternberg, Predicting antigen presentation-what could we learn from a million peptides? Frontiers in Immunology 9 (2018) 1716. Available from: https://doi.org/10.3389/fimmu.2018.01716. Published 2018 Jul 25.
[8] J.A. Traherne, Human MHC architecture and evolution: implications for disease association studies, International Journal of Immunogenetics 35 (3) (2008) 179–192. Available from: https://doi.org/10.1111/j.1744-313X.2008.00765.x.
[9] V. Matzaraki, V. Kumar, C. Wijmenga, A. Zhernakova, The MHC locus and genetic susceptibility to autoimmune and infectious diseases, Genome Biology 18 (1) (2017) 76. Available from: https://doi.org/10.1186/s13059-017-1207-1. Published 2017 Apr 27.
[10] K.L. Rock, E. Reits, J. Neefjes, Present yourself! By MHC class I and MHC class II molecules, Trends in Immunology 37 (11) (2016) 724–737. Available from: https://doi.org/10.1016/j.it.2016.08.010.
[11] H. Luo, H. Ye, H.W. Ng, et al., Machine learning methods for predicting HLA-peptide binding activity, Bioinformatics and Biology Insights 9 (Suppl. 3) (2015) 21–29. Available from: https://doi.org/10.4137/BBI.S29466. Published 2015 Oct 11.
[12] A. Szaflarska, M. Rutkowska-Zapała, D. Kowalczyk, Krótka charakterystyka mechanizmów tolerancji immunologicznej [Immune tolerance mechanisms–brief review], Przeglad Lekarski 72 (12) (2015) 765–769.
[13] A. Doria, M. Zen, S. Bettio, et al., Autoinflammation and autoimmunity: bridging the divide, Autoimmunity Reviews 12 (1) (2012) 22–30. Available from: https://doi.org/10.1016/j.autrev.2012.07.018.
[14] D. Qi, E. Wu, Cancer prognosis: considering tumor and its microenvironment as a whole, EBioMedicine 43 (2019) 28–29. Available from: https://doi.org/10.1016/j.ebiom.2019.04.031.
[15] T. Blankenstein, P.G. Coulie, E. Gilboa, E.M. Jaffee, The determinants of tumour immunogenicity, Nature Reviews Cancer 12 (4) (2012) 307–313. Available from: https://doi.org/10.1038/nrc3246. Published 2012 Mar 1.
[16] H. Gonzalez, C. Hagerling, Z. Werb, Roles of the immune system in cancer: from tumor initiation to metastatic progression, Genes & Development 32 (19–20) (2018) 1267–1284. Available from: https://doi.org/10.1101/gad.314617.118.
[17] D. Ostroumov, N. Fekete-Drimusz, M. Saborowski, F. Kühnel, N. Woller, CD4 and CD8 T lymphocyte interplay in controlling tumor growth, Cellular and Molecular Life Sciences: CMLS 75 (4) (2018) 689–713. Available from: https://doi.org/10.1007/s00018-017-2686-7.

[18] P. Mahdavi Sharif, P. Jabbari, S. Razi, M. Keshavarz-Fathi, N. Rezaei, Importance of TNF-alpha and its alterations in the development of cancers [published online ahead of print, 2020 Mar 21], Cytokine 130 (2020) 155066. Available from: https://doi.org/10.1016/j.cyto.2020.155066.
[19] J.S. O'Donnell, M.W.L. Teng, M.J. Smyth, Cancer immunoediting and resistance to T cell-based immunotherapy, Nature Reviews Clinical Oncology 16 (3) (2019) 151–167. Available from: https://doi.org/10.1038/s41571-018-0142-8.
[20] J.J. Wang, K.F. Lei, F. Han, Tumor microenvironment: recent advances in various cancer treatments, European Review for Medical and Pharmacological Sciences 22 (12) (2018) 3855–3864. Available from: https://doi.org/10.26355/eurrev_201806_15270.
[21] V. Schirrmacher, From chemotherapy to biological therapy: a review of novel concepts to reduce the side effects of systemic cancer treatment (review), International Journal of Oncology 54 (2) (2019) 407–419. Available from: https://doi.org/10.3892/ijo.2018.4661.

CHAPTER

2

Introduction to bioinformatics

What is bioinformatics?

Over the past few decades, advancements in computer sciences have taken the world in their stride. In every branch of science, computers help scientists in every aspect, from collection and manipulation of data to their visualization, making predictions, and simulations, among others. There is virtually no aspect of science that computers cannot help with.

Biologists, studying the living organisms and discovering new aspects of life, are no exception. Before the era of high-throughput technology, observations of biologists would lead to the generation of data that were relatively small in volume. These data could be easily stored on a computer and manipulated using simple mathematics and principal statistical models.

However, emergence of new technologies that enabled biologists study the living organisms to their finest core changed the requirements for mastering biology [1]. To elaborate the integration of life sciences with high-throughput technology and data handling, let us go through an example. Imagine having a picture from an analog camera at hand and writing the details you see from this picture on a notebook. While holding the printed picture, you cannot see the minutest details and the notebook seems to be more than adequate to place all the details you see. Now imagine you have the same picture on a computer. You can zoom in on every detail and analyze each section of the picture. This will indeed lead to the generation of a wealth of information, which cannot fit into a notebook. So you decide to create files on your computer to write these details down. As technology improves, you can take a more vivid picture and will be able to see more details. Now you will probably need to store the information you get from each section of the picture in a different file on your computer. The same has happened with biology. Before the high-throughput technology, biologists' observations were not detailed, and many aspects of molecular

Immunoinformatics of Cancers
DOI: https://doi.org/10.1016/B978-0-12-822400-7.00011-7

interaction were not discovered. However, once high-throughput technology helped us study different pathways in a living organism, biology branched into new disciplines such as metabolomics, genomics, proteomics, lipidomics, glycomics, etc. [2]. These -omics are like different sections of the picture we were holding in our hand. Every day, new pathways and details are discovered in each of these -omics, which calls for the creation of spaces that can hold this information and new tools to manipulate them so that they can make sense in respect to the living organism. This way these technologies help us move toward the ultimate goal of personalized medicine.

In the example of discovering new details of a picture, creating new files in our computer to store the data collected from our observations translates into creating databases storing the high volume of data gained from studying living organisms [1]. Currently, there are many online databases serving the purpose of storage and distribution of the data collected from observations with high-throughput technologies. On the other hand, there are many tools to manipulate these data, many of which are online and free resources offered by the same databases. The novel technologies of studying different mechanisms in an organism, the databases that store the data obtained from using such technologies, and the knowledge of recruiting studies are the mainstay of bioinformatics. Many of these databases are curated in an omics-based fashion. Some of the most practical databases in the field of immunoinformatics are introduced in Chapter 3.

In this chapter, we will briefly overview the most important concepts of the immunoinformatics.

Immunoinformatics

Immunology, as a major field of biology, is no exception to what was mentioned earlier regarding its integration with high-throughput technologies and novel computational tools. In Chapter 1, the role of the immune system in infectious diseases and malignancies as well as other disorders was briefly discussed. However, thanks to the advances of the technology in probing pathways of many physiologic and pathologic interactions in organisms, we now know that the immune system has a much broader role in organisms. Research on immunology has focused on multi-omics of this system [3]. The multi-omics, at a single-cell level, organism level, and population level, have broadened our knowledge regarding the "immunomics," the study of all aspects of the immunome, which are all the genes and proteins that play a role in the immune system [4]. The -omics most relatable to the immunomics seem to be genomics, transcriptomics, and proteomics [3,5]. However, ongoing investigations have shed light on the role of other -omics, such as metabolomics, in the immune system. The immune system has close interactions with the metabolism of organisms. For instance, defects in metabolism can lead to immunodeficiencies. On the other hand, the immune system can control the absorption of nutrients from the intestinal mucosa and affect the metabolism [5]. Therefore, the interactions of immune system and metabolism, if we choose to see them as distinct systems, affects the physiology of many systems within the organism.

Immunoinformatics not only helps with storing and analyzing the data created by research in multi-omics of the immune system, but also enables immunologists to perform in silico studies [6,7]. One of the good examples of recruiting in silico studies to advance immunological studies is the case of using the in silico models to predict the immunogenicity of the epitopes and designing new vaccines [6,7]. This can be considered as a more ethical and cost-effective approach to developing new therapeutics. The knowledge gained from these studies can be implemented in in vitro studies [8]. For these reasons, many databases and algorithms are dedicated to the epitomics, which is the study of epitope interactions with antigen receptors, major histocompatibility complex (MHC) molecules, and antibodies [9]. Advances in epitomics, as well as in many other aspects of the immunoinformatics, are indebted to the high-throughput technologies, which are evolving rapidly in response to the need for more accurate and accelerated methods to study molecular aspects of living organisms.

High-throughput technologies

Microarray

Many advances in techniques have been made to study the interactions within the MHC–peptide–T cell complexes as well as the genomics, epigenomics, proteomics, and transcriptomics of the immune system. Many of them are based on microarray techniques. Microarray was one of the first high-throughput techniques used to reveal expression levels of a few to hundreds of thousands of genes or proteins at the same time [10]. The basis of microarray studies is hybridization of biological molecules [11]. Microarrays have various implementations in immunologic studies, from gene expression and methylation to antibody microarrays (antibody arrays), which study the binding of antibodies to specific antigens.

There are several commercial microarray chips designed to conduct different studies. In these chips, there are thousands of micro-level wells. In each well, there is a very small amount of DNA sequence of a particular gene or a collection of proteins (e.g., antibodies). These DNA sequences or proteins fixed on a solid surface, such as silicon, plastic, or glass, are called *probes*. Each microarray chip, which is commercially prepared, has as many tiny wells as the number of the specific probes. In DNA microarray studies, messenger RNA (mRNA) of different genes from experiment and control groups are extracted. Complementary DNA (cDNA) of these mRNA samples, which are representative of the transcriptome of experiment and control groups, respectively, are generated and labeled with fluorescent tags of two different colors. These cDNA molecules then bind the probes in each well in a competitive manner, a process known as hybridization. After hybridization, the microarray chip is scanned for fluorescent reflection. If a well appears to be of the color representing the experiment group, the gene assigned to that well is expressed more in the experiment group. If the expression of a particular gene is equal in both the experiment and the control groups, the color of that well appears as a color between the two fluorescent tags. Fig. 2.1 explains the DNA microarray technique. Protein microarray techniques can help with epitope mapping. The information obtained from these studies will provide the basics of epitope prediction for in silico studies.

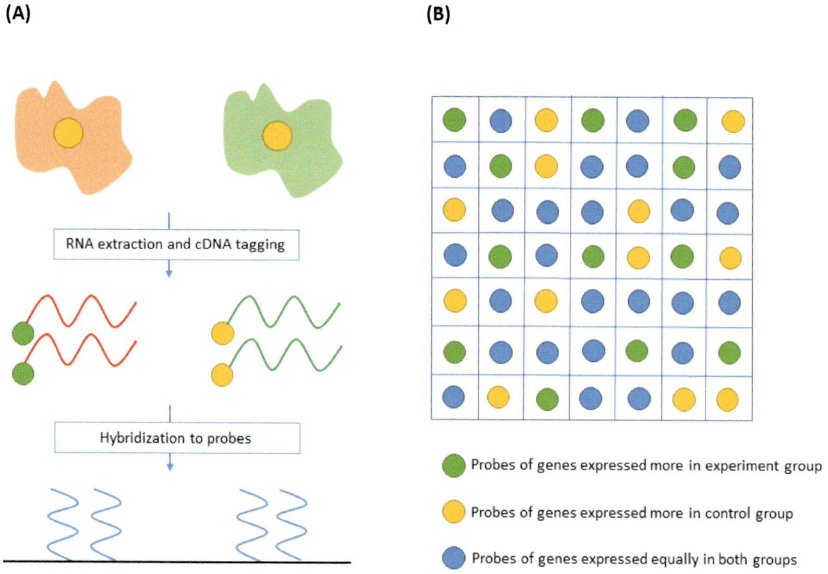

FIGURE 2.1 Basics of DNA microarray. (A) mRNA is extracted from experiment and control tissue, complementary DNA (cDNA) is made from these mRNAs and tagged with different fluorescent colors. These cDNA strands hybridize with commercially prepared probes. (B) Wells in which probes hybridize more with DNA of the experiment group appear as the color of the experiment group (*green* in this picture), and those that hybridize equally with the DNA of the experiment group and the control group, appear as a mixture of both fluorescent colors (*blue* in this picture).

Computers and biological data

Developments in biological techniques are made in parallel with the progress of computer sciences. In fact, we owe many of the current biological techniques to computers. Computers can perform complicated analyses at high speed and accuracy. These analyses have provided a vast majority of the curated data we have at hand today, such as a complete genome of several organisms, gene functions, etc. Computational methods serve immunological studies in various aspects. The first use of computers and computational modeling can be traced back to the modeling of malaria epidemiology [12]. Computers can also be used to model the immune response to different pathogenic phenomena, such as allergens, infection, and cancer. In many cases, this requires epitope prediction, an important and challenging area of immunoinformatics [13].

Epitope predictions are different for B cells and T cells and they have their own complexities [13]. Epitopes of B cells are usually conformational, which means they cannot be directly inferred from the peptide sequence, unless the spatial conformation of that peptide is retrieved from its sequence [14]. Machine learning approaches help with retrieving the peptide conformation from its sequence. On the other hand, epitope mapping for T cells requires determining the anchor motif for class I and II MHC molecules. Several databases are dedicated to B cell and T cell epitope prediction, and many of them offer online tools for making these predictions [14]. Some of these databases are described in Chapter 3.

Epitope prediction and antigen presentation are of utmost importance in designing therapeutic agents such as vaccines for either infection diseases or cancers [15]. Some tumor-associated antigens have known epitopes for T cells, which are available online and can be used to predict immune responses against cancers. Furthermore, these antigens can be used to design monoclonal antibodies (mAbs) or chimeric antigen receptor T cells against cancers exhibiting these specific antigens. How immune system responds to these antigens can be predicted through models simulating the immune system responses [15]. Even though the reliability of the findings from in silico studies are increasing, an important point to bear in mind regarding the in silico interactions of the immune system is to actually test them through experiments.

References

[1] V. D'Argenio, The high-throughput analyses era: are we ready for the data struggle? High Throughput 7 (1) (2018) 8.

[2] X. Yang, R. Jiao, L. Yang, L.P. Wu, Y.R. Li, J. Wang, C. Yi, 33 (8) (2011) 829–846.

[3] J. Yu, J. Peng, H. Chi, Systems immunology: integrating multi-omics data to infer regulatory networks and hidden drivers of immunity, Current Opinion in Systems Biology 15 (2019) 19–29.

[4] A.S. De Groot, Immunome-derived vaccines, Expert Opinion on Biological Therapy 4 (6) (2004) 767–772.
[5] D.C. Nieman, M.A. Lila, N.D. Gillitt, Immunometabolism: a multi-omics approach to interpreting the influence of exercise and diet on the immune system, Annual Review of Food Science and Technology 10 (2019) 341–363.
[6] A.A. Bahrami, Z. Payandeh, S. Khalili, A. Zakeri, M. Bandehpour, Immunoinformatics: in silico approaches and computational design of a multi-epitope, immunogenic protein, International Reviews of Immunology 38 (6) (2019) 307–322.
[7] N. Hajighahramani, N. Nezafat, M. Eslami, M. Negahdaripour, S.S. Rahmatabadi, Y. Ghasemi, Immunoinformatics analysis and in silico designing of a novel multi-epitope peptide vaccine against *Staphylococcus aureus*, Infection, Genetics and Evolution 48 (2017) 83–94.
[8] M.E. Oraiopoulou, E. Tzamali, G. Tzedakis, et al., Integrating in vitro experiments with in silico approaches for Glioblastoma invasion: the role of cell-to-cell adhesion heterogeneity, Scientific Reports 8 (1) (2018) 16200.
[9] P. Jabbari, N. Rezaei, Artificial intelligence and immunotherapy, Expert Review of Clinical Immunology 15 (7) (2019) 689–691.
[10] Z. Chen, T. Dodig-Crnković, J.M. Schwenk, S.C. Tao, Current applications of antibody microarrays, Clinical Proteomics 15 (2018) 7.
[11] R. Bumgarner, Overview of DNA microarrays: types, applications, and their future, Current Protocols in Molecular Biology (2013). Available from: https://doi.org/10.1002/0471142727.mb2201s101. Edited by Frederick M. Ausubel ... [et al.]; Chapter 22: Unit-22. 1.
[12] R. Ross, An application of the theory of probabilities to the study ofa prioripathometry. Part I, Proceedings of the Royal Society of London. Series A92 (1916) 204–230.
[13] J.C. Tong, E.C. Ren, Immunoinformatics: current trends and future directions, Drug Discovery Today 14 (13–14) (2009) 684–689.
[14] J.L. Sanchez-Trincado, M. Gomez-Perosanz, P.A. Reche, Fundamentals and methods for T- and B-cell epitope prediction, Journal of Immunology Research 2017 (2017) 2680160.
[15] S. Draghici, M. Chatterjee, M.A. Tainsky, Epitomics: serum screening for the early detection of cancer on microarrays using complex panels of tumor antigens, Expert Review of Molecular Diagnostics 5 (5) (2005) 735–743.

CHAPTER

3

Practical databases and online tools in immunoinformatics

Introduction

As mentioned in the previous chapter, one of the most important aspects of bioinformatics is the database that stores and provides a wealth of information generated from the biological studies. Some of these databases already hold petabytes (10^{15} bytes) of data, and this number is increasing as you are reading this book. The Human Genome Project (HGP), which started in 1990 and completed in 2003, has generated more data than individual biology experiments or projects [1]. The information from this project increases as we bring into account the variations among individuals. Furthermore, the current trend in the use of high-throughput experiments such as microarray expression profiling, RNA sequencing, Chromatin Immunoprecipitation Sequencing (ChIP-Seq), and genome-wide association studies (GWAS) produces large amounts of data, which need to be curated and properly stored for use by researchers. There are numerous databases available for the storage of such information [2]. Each of these databases has a unique characteristic that demarcates it form other databases. However, some of them are quite similar, with the only difference being they are managed by different institutes or organizations. As an example, Gene Expression Omnibus (GEO) (http://www.ncbi.nlm.nih.gov/geo/) is a genomic data repository affiliated to the National Center for Biotechnology Information (NCBI), which archives and provides information regarding the expression profile of genes. ArrayExpress (http://www.ebi.ac.uk/arrayexpress/) and Expression Atlas are similar functional genomics repositories affiliated to The European Bioinformatics Institute (EMBL-EBI). Therefore, the data archived in such similar databases have a major overlap.

Immunoinformatics of Cancers
DOI: https://doi.org/10.1016/B978-0-12-822400-7.00005-1

An important topic of study for immunoinformatics is the B cell and T cell epitope prediction, for which there are many databases, algorithms, and online tools available. There are many more databases available dealing with allergens, autoimmune diseases, and viral agents, which are beyond the scope of this book. In this chapter, we will introduce some of the most important databases and repositories required for research in immunoinformatics.

ImMunoGeneTics information system

The ImMunoGeneTics (IMGT) information system (http://imgt.org/) can be considered as an interface between immunogenetics and bioinformatics. IMGT is the first immunoinformatics database created and can be regarded as the encyclopedia of immunoinformatics [3]. It was founded in 1989, and this repository archives variable (V), diversity (D), joining (J), and constant (C) genes, which enabled studying the adaptive immune responses and their diversity from a genomics perspective through its interactive tools. This repository includes many databases, online tools, and Web resources. IMGT archives data related to the immune system of humans and other vertebrates, and the databases of this repository are divided into four categories: sequence databases, genome databases, structure databases, and monoclonal antibodies databases. Genomics and proteomics of virtually all components of the immune system such as immunoglobulins, T cell receptors, major histocompatibility superfamilies as well as other proteins related to the immune system such as therapeutic monoclonal antibodies can be found in this database. Data are organized and retrievable by the IGMT-ONTOLOGY system based on seven axioms: IDENTIFICATION, DESCRIPTION, CLASSIFICATION, NUMEROTATION, LOCALIZATION, ORIENTATION, and OBTENTION, which results in more accurate and easier search strategies.

Immune epitope database

This database (http://www.iedb.org) catalogs experimental data on antibody and T cell epitopes studied in several species, including humans, other primates, mouse, and fish [4]. The database has a user-friendly interface, which allows an efficient search of information on peptidic epitopes of more than 1 million entries on the database. In addition to storing information regarding epitopes of antigens, this database can be used as a tool for predicting the binding of epitopes with different classes of major histocompatibility complex (MHC).

Cancer antigenic peptide database

This database (https://caped.icp.ucl.ac.be) stores curated information on cancer-specific epitopes [5]. This database is one of the many databases of its kind storing information on cancer antigens and epitopes. These databases are very important in cancer research as they provide information on antigens that are appropriate candidates for vaccine development.

In this database, antigens are curated into different categories based on factors such as their mutation, specification to a tumor, etc. The antigens are linked to GeneCards (https://www.genecards.org) for more information, and complementary information regarding each antigen is provided in the database. Furthermore, candidate peptides with their comprehensive characterization are stored in a complementary section, but these peptides lack the complementary information provided for other definite peptides.

NEPdb: a database of T-cell experimentally-validated neoantigens and pan-cancer predicted neoepitopes for cancer immunotherapy

Similar to the Cancer Antigen Peptide Database, this database is an important tool for the immunotherapy of cancers. This database has curated more than 17,000 validated human immunogenic and nonimmunogenic neoepitope entries with human leukocyte antigens and T cell details that have been curated from published literature [6]. In addition to presenting effective cancer-associated neoantigens, this database also delineates which neoantigens are not potent cancer-associated antigens for immunotherapy. However, a shortcoming of this database, as is evident by its name, is that it does not include all cancer-associated antigens.

There are more prospective cancer antigen and epitope databases, such as the the Cancer Epitope Database and Analysis Resource (CEDAR) [5]. Such comprehensive epitope databases and analysis tools are important for the development of effective cancer immunotherapies. Before overviewing online immunoinformatics tools, we introduce two important databases in the field of bioinformatics: GEO and The Cancer Genome Atlas (TCGA). Even though these databases are not confined to immunoinformatics, it is important for researchers in the field of bioinformatics to have fair knowledge of these databases.

Gene expression omnibus

GEO is a public database of high-throughput experiments on gene expression in which data from various methods of gene expression such as hybridization-based (e.g., microarray) and synthesis-based (e.g., RNA sequencing) methods are deposited. This database is a part of NCBI. As mentioned earlier, there are other European databases similar to this database, ArrayExpress and Expression Atlas. There are more than 4000 datasets in the GEO repository, which encompass more than 150,000 series and nearly 5 million samples. Many datasets deposited in this repository are readily available to all researchers in various formats.

In addition to providing expression profiles, GEO has a strong and practical analysis tool for expression by array profiles, called GEO2R. "GEO2R is an interactive web tool that allows users to compare two or more groups of Samples in a GEO Series in order to identify genes that are differentially expressed across experimental conditions." In Chapter 16, we will be using data from this database to make predictive models.

The cancer genome atlas

Even though TCGA can be considered as a database as cancer-related data in different formats can be retrieved from it, it is basically a project jointly managed by the National Cancer Institute and the National Human Genome Research Institute. The aim of this program is to discover and curate cancer-causing mutations and genetic factors [7]. Thus far, TCGA has "generated over 2.5 petabytes of genomic, epigenomic, transcriptomic, and proteomic data."

In addition to providing genomic, epigenomic, transcriptomic, and proteomic data, this program provides several online interactive tools and software packages for the analysis of various data retrieved from TCGA. These tools and software have user manuals and workflows to help users navigate them. In addition, there are several online guidelines and resources that can be used for retrieving data from TCGA and analyzing them using its associated tools and software, which are beyond the scope of this book.

Online immunoinformatics tools

In addition to the tools and software introduced before, we overview an example of free online tools on the prediction of MHC–peptide binding and conformation of epitopes, two of the most important topics in immunoinformatics. There are numerous predictive models that have been developed for this purpose using different machine learning algorithms, hoping to outperform other algorithms in their accuracy. Some of these models are available to all researchers through online databases and tools; however, some are merely published work and not available in large scales.

EpiSearch: mapping of conformational epitopes

EpiSearch is one of the free online tools that allow prediction of epitopes based on the peptide sequence and protein data bank files. In order to predict epitopes, first, a three-dimensional structure of the peptide is predicted. The basis of predictions for EpiSearch is similar to that of immune epitope database (IEDB) epitope_MHC binding prediction [8]. The algorithms behind this tool are trained based on experimentally observed conformational epitopes by X-ray crystallography.

Immune epitope database epitope–MHC binding prediction tools

One of the most easily accessible online prediction tools for predicting MHC-I and MHC-II binding to epitopes is the IEDB prediction tool. In this interactive tool, users can provide their peptide sequence, choose the type of MHC they want to assay, and the organism in which MHC–peptide binding is being predicted. These tools use machine learning algorithms such as position-specific scoring matrix, support vector machine, and support vector regression along with other machine learning algorithms [9].

In addition to these free online tools, there are several software and commercial online tools available that allow prediction of protein structure and MHC–peptide binding. Details of these tools and published predictive models are beyond the scope of this book. In the future chapters, we focus on the basics of machine learning to create our own predictive models using example and real-world data.

References

[1] L. Hood, L. Rowen, The Human Genome Project: big science transforms biology and medicine, Genome Medicine 5 (9) (2013) 79. Available from: https://doi.org/10.1186/gm483.

[2] D. Zou, L. Ma, J. Yu, Z. Zhang, Biological databases for human research, Genomics, Proteomics & Bioinformatics 13 (1) (2015) 55–63. Available from: https://doi.org/10.1016/j.gpb.2015.01.006.

[3] M.P. Lefranc, V. Giudicelli, Q. Kaas, E. Duprat, J. Jabado-Michaloud, D. Scaviner, et al., IMGT, the international ImMunoGeneTics information system, Nucleic Acids Research 33 (Database issue) (2005) D593–D597. https://doi.org/10.1093.

[4] R. Vita, S. Mahajan, J.A. Overton, S.K. Dhanda, S. Martini, J.R. Cantrell, et al., The immune epitope database (IEDB): 2018 update, Nucleic Acids Research 47 (D1) (2019) D339–D343. Available from: https://doi.org/10.1093/nar/gky1006.

[5] Z. Koşaloğlu-Yalçın, N. Blazeska, H. Carter, M. Nielsen, E. Cohen, D. Kufe, et al., The cancer epitope database and analysis resource: a blueprint for the establishment of a new bioinformatics resource for use by the cancer immunology community, Frontiers in Immunology 12 (2021) 735609. Available from: https://doi.org/10.3389/fimmu.2021.735609.

[6] J. Xia, P. Bai, W. Fan, Q. Li, Y. Li, D. Wang, et al., NEPdb: a database of T-cell experimentally-validated neoantigens and pan-cancer predicted neoepitopes for cancer immunotherapy, Frontiers in Immunology 12 (2021) 644637. Available from: https://doi.org/10.3389/fimmu.2021.644637.

[7] K. Tomczak, P. Czerwińska, M. Wiznerowicz, The Cancer Genome Atlas (TCGA): an immeasurable source of knowledge, Contemporary Oncology (Poznan, Poland) 19 (1A) (2015) A68–A77. Available from: https://doi.org/10.5114/wo.2014.47136.

[8] H. Luo, H. Ye, H.W. Ng, L. Shi, W. Tong, D.L. Mendrick, et al., Machine learning methods for predicting HLA-peptide binding activity, Bioinformatics and Biology Insights 9 (Suppl. 3) (2015) 21–29. Available from: https://doi.org/10.4137/BBI.S29466.

[9] S.S. Negi, W. Braun, Automated detection of conformational epitopes using phage display Peptide sequences, Bioinformatics and Biology Insights 3 (2009) 71–81. Available from: https://doi.org/10.4137/bbi.s2745.

SECTION II

Basics of R programming

CHAPTER

4

Principles of programming in R

What is R?

R refers to an open source programming language as well as a development environment used for developing applications for scientific calculation, data manipulation, and efficient graphical display. It can be considered as an implementation of the S language, which was developed prior to R. Some consider the R programming language hard to learn, but there are many advantageous points about R that makes it easy to implement and a favorite programming environment for biologists. There are different packages developed for the R environment, which makes it easier to employ R. The packages give R powerful graphical display tools, which might be considered the best for graphical display of data. Also, there are many third-party graphical user interfaces (GUIs) for R, the most widely known being RStudio, which makes programming in the R environment even easier.

Every year, there have been releases of two versions of the R environment. The latest version of R can be download from `http://www.r-project.org/` or from the several mirrors that belong to the Comprehensive R Archive Network (CRAN) at `http://cran.r-project.org/mirrors.html`.

There are different repositories for R in which packages are stored. The most important packages for programming in the R environment, which will be useful for bioinformaticians, will be introduced in Chapter 6.

What is RStudio?

As mentioned earlier, RStudio is one of the third-party GUIs or an integrated development environment (IDE) available for R; however,

DOI: https://doi.org/10.1016/B978-0-12-822400-7.00003-8

it also works well with other programming languages, such as Python. For many reasons, programming in a GUI is preferred. Coding is in general easier in these interfaces as they decrease the chances of syntax errors. Furthermore, they can provide higher quality graphics as well as a more esthetic working space. Even though some limitations may be faced when using such interfaces, we prefer using RStudio as our programming environment in this book. RStudio can be freely downloaded at `https://rstudio.com/products/rstudio/download/`. Note that RStudio is based on R; therefore R must be downloaded and installed before RStudio is installed.

RStudio working environment

Now that you have RStudio installed in your device, you can see that there are four windows (panes) in the default view (Fig. 4.1). You can modify their position in the program environment; however, in the original view, on the top left is the "source" window. You can write you codes in this space without actually running them and can also go back to your codes to edit them and save them for future use. Just like opening new tabs in an internet browser, you can create a new source window by pressing `shift + ctrl + N`, if you are a Windows user, or `shift + command (cmd) +` N on Mac. In order to run the code line(s), select the line(s) and then click `alt + enter` or `ctrl + enter` or click "Run" at the top right-hand side of the "source" window. The window at the bottom left-hand side is the "console." This is where running codes

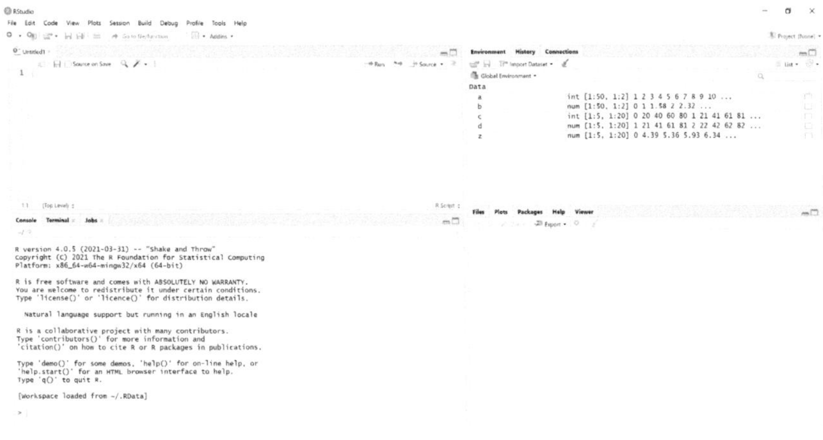

FIGURE 4.1 The default view of RStudio, an Integrated Development Environment for R.

appear and will be evaluated by R. You cannot edit the written codes in "console" as easily as you edit them in "source"; however, by pressing "Page up," previous lines of code will be retrieved, which you can edit based on the errors you get from R. The window at the top right-hand side is the "Environment/History" window. All objects that you have created in R will appear in this window, which will provide you with an ability to quickly review your objects and their characteristics. The "History" window will store all the commands ever ran in R. From the same window, you can import data from different software such as Excel, SPSS, Stata, etc. The window at the bottom right-hand side displays the list of installed packages, plots, and the files on your device. You can also set your "working directory" (explained below) from this window. The "Help" menu for RStudio explains the functions, arguments, etc., in the Viewer window, and data frames and other rectangular data sets are also shown.

Some points to remember about R

Before getting started with R, there are a few important points to learn about R that will always hold true. Firstly, we must make sure that R is ready to receive commands from us. How R indicates that? By displaying the R prompt, which is the character ">." If the R prompt is not shown in the R console, check for any running or incomplete commands and fix it.

The inputs you give R for the first time must always be placed inside " " or ' ' , as if you are introducing your input to R. Once your input has been introduced to R, you can call it without " " or ' '. An example of such inputs is when we install new packages. We will discuss this through examples later in this chapter.

If you are preparing an R script in your "Source" window, it is recommended to put comments at different stages of preparing the script by using the pound sign (#). R knows that what follows a "#" does not count as a command or operation and it will not run it, but this way your script will be easier to follow for others who might use it or for your future reference. Throughout this chapter and the future chapters, we will be referring to some of the additional comments using the pound (£) sign, for the sake of practice.

A point to remember, which has the potential to ensnare even the experts in programming, is that R is case sensitive. Be careful about the inputs you give to R with capital letters, which must always be called with capital letters and vice versa. Another example of a simple, yet mazing point is employing round brackets in R. At times our commands and inputs have a complicated structure in which many brackets are used. Each opening parenthesis must have a corresponding closing parenthesis. One way to make sure of this is by clicking on each parenthesis, which will highlight the corresponding opening or closing parenthesis, and if the corresponding parenthesis is missing, we can add it.

When working with R, you must indicate your "working directory." Your working directory is where R will look for data and files in your device. Your default working directory is usually your home directory. In order to know what your working directory is, run the command `getwd()` (get working directory). If you prefer organizing your data in a way that will need a different working directory, simply change it using the command `setwd()`. There is also a hard way of choosing the working directory by typing the complete address of the location we want R to look for data and files. However, there are also easier ways to choose the working directory: if the operating system of your device is Windows, you can open your file, copy the address from the address bar, and paste it inside the in your command. However, remember that all slashes must be converted into backslashes. For Mac users, this conversion is not needed.

Example:

```
> getwd()

[1] "C:/Users/Immunoinformatics/Documents"

#changing the working directory by copying address from address bar
and converting "\" to "/"

> setwd("C:/Users/Immunoinformatics/Desktop/Data")
```

Note that the address is placed inside the as you are introducing it to R for the first time.

There is also an easier way of changing the working directory. Once you type the command `setwd()`, press the Tab button to choose the new working directory.

R repositories

Repositories are vehicles that R uses to distribute and organize packages. There are different repositories in R, which contain package tar files. Each package is available through a certain R repository.

Some repositories are essential in the field of bioinformatics due to the packages that are frequently used in this field. Like packages that must be "called" in each new R session, repositories must be selected in each session. A list of repositories can be obtained through the command `setRepositories()`:

```
> setRepositories()
--- Please select repositories for use in this session ---


1: + CRAN
2:   BioC software
3:   BioC annotation
4:   BioC experiment
5:   CRAN (extras)
6:   Omegahat
7:   R-Forge
8:   rforge.net
```

You can see that CRAN, as the main R repository, is already selected. You can also note that R waits for you to enter the number of repositories you would like R to select from, and the console will not be ready to receive new commands until you enter the number of repositories.

```
Enter one or more numbers separated by spaces, or an empty line to cancel
1:
```

You can select all the repositories by typing numbers 2–8 (with a space between numbers); however, the first four repositories support most of the packages in the field of bioinformatics.

```
1: 2 3 4
```

If we get the list of repositories again, then we can see that the corresponding repositories have been selected.

```
> setRepositories()
--- Please select repositories for use in this session ---


1: + CRAN
2: + BioC software
3: + BioC annotation
4: + BioC experiment
5:   CRAN (extras)
6:   Omegahat
7:   R-Forge
8:   rforge.net
```

Getting packages in R

As mentioned before, predeveloped packages provide R users with easy-to-implement functions. There are many packages developed for different purposes, which we need to install in R before using them. In order to install packages, use the command `install.packages()`. What you type inside the round brackets, they must be placed inside a as this is the first time you are mentioning this name in the R environment. It is like introducing the name of the package to R. As an example, let us install the package `ggplot2`, as it is one of the most widely used packages developed for R.

```
> install.packages("ggplot2")
```

Once you have installed a certain package, it will remain in your R environment for ever. However, in order to be able to implement the package, we must "call" the package every time we open a new R session. We can call the packages by using either of the following commands (note that you do not need to place the name of the package inside to call it):

```
> require(ggplot2) #or by the library() function
> library(ggplot2)
```

Updating R

As mentioned before, each year two updates of R are released. There are different ways to get these updates. An easy way for Windows users to get those updates is through using the following commands:

```
> install.packages ("installr")
> installr :: updateR ()
```

You can also update your R environment and downloaded packages to the latest version available by going to Tools > Check for Package Updates. . . .

Getting help in R

There are three ways to ask R for help regarding functions, classes, data sets, and objects. The `help()` function will provide access to the documentation of what is written inside the parentheses (with or without). In order to access documentations regarding a function in a package that is not loaded, we need to specify the package through using the command `help(FunctionName, package = "PackageName")`. Another way to access the documentations is through the "?" operator; for example, the `?matrix` will get you to the corresponding documentations.

The basic functions and operations

R can be considered a powerful calculator as it runs various complicated operations. Table 4.1 summarizes some of the operators, their meaning in the R environment as well as simple examples of how to implement them:

TABLE 4.1 Operators in R.

Operator	Meaning and function	Example
[	Indexing, getting a subset of an object	> LETTERS[1] [1] "A"
[[	Indexing, getting one special element out of an object	> iris[["Petal.Length"]]
$	Indexing, for accessing an element by its exact name	> iris$Petal.Length
+ -	Add and subtract	> 1 + 2 [1] 3
/ *	Divide and multiply	> 2*1 [1] 2
^	Exponentiation (right to left)	> 3^2 [1] 9
< > == != >= =<	Comparison and ordering	> 2 + 1! = 3 [1] FALSE
->> = ->	Assignment	> a = 2 + 3 > a [1] 5

Note: LETTERS is a built-in vector of the 26 uppercase letters of the Roman alphabet. iris is another built-in data set regarding certain traits of iris.

NOTE

When working in R environment, you may get certain notes from the program, highlighted in red. These notes are mostly either a warning message or an error. In the case of warning messages, you do not need to worry, as the program is only providing you with some additional information and it runs the command successfully. However, in the case of an error, the program cannot run the command and instead, provides feedback through the errors on how to resolve the issues that prevented it from running the command.

Assignment and variables

A variable can be considered a memory location where we store values. Once you assign a value or result of a computation to a variable, it will remain so until you assign a new value to that variable. For example:

```
#assign the result of an operation to the variable "A"
> A=2+1
> A
[1] 3
```

Every time we call "A," the returned value will be "3," until we assign a new value to it.

Objects and classes

In the example above, "A" is an object of the "numeric" class. Objects can be of simple or more complex structures, based on their class. The "class" is the data type in which R stores objects. There are several classes in R; we will review some of them that are most commonly used in bioinformatics.

Numeric objects

In the example above, we assigned a numeric value to "A." On asking R about the class of "A," it will return "numeric":

```
> class(A)
[1] "numeric"
```

Character objects

Characters are used to store "string" values in R. String values are text in nature, that is, they include characters as opposed to numbers. The following examples represent some structures of "character" objects:

```
> B= "immunoinformatics"
> B
[1] "immunoinformatics"
> class(B)
[1] "character"
```

Another way to create a "vector" of character strings is to combine them using the concatenate (c) function:

```
> C=c("immunology", 1, "bioinformatics")
> class(C)
[1] "character"
```

A "vector" is an array of values of the same class. In the example above, vector C includes a numeric value of "1"; however, the class of this value will be character, like the rest of values:

```
> class(C[2])
[1] "character"
```

There are other classes of variables such as "logical" variables, which are the result of comparisons. As an example:

```
> is.integer(C[2])
[1] FALSE
```

Factor variables

Factor variables are categorical variables and can be character or numeric in nature. Factor variables are important in terms of machine learning and classification of data (Chapter 10). Saving your string variables as factors is more efficient in terms of memory and time consumption for developing our model. In the data set below, the third column corresponds to the targeted tumor-associated antigens (TAAs). The three classes of TAAs are three "levels" of the factor variable "target TAA":

```
> data
   Gender Age target.TAA Survival.mo.
1       1  59    IL13R?2            6
2       1  63   EGFRvIII            5
3       2  71    IL13R?2           12
4       1  67      CD133            4
5       2  48   EGFRvIII           10
6       1  78      CD133            6
7       1  65    IL13R?2            5
8       2  65    IL13R?2            7
9       1  73   EGFRvIII            2
10      2  78   EGFRvIII           NA
11      1  56    IL13R?2           14
12      1  67      CD133            7
13      2  69      CD133            9
14      2  43    IL13R?2            6
15      2  58   EGFRvIII           NA
16      1  61      CD133            3
17      1  60    IL13R?2            5
18      2  75   EGFRvIII           13
19      2  66   EGFRvIII            7
20      1  56      CD133           NA
```

We check the class of the third column in the data set:

```
> class(data[,3])
[1] "factor"
```

```
> data[,3]
 [1] IL13Ra2  EGFRvIII IL13Ra2  CD133    EGFRvIII CD133    IL13Ra2  IL13Ra2
     EGFRvIII EGFRvIII IL13Ra2  CD133    CD133    IL13Ra2  EGFRvIII CD133
[17] IL13Ra2  EGFRvIII EGFRvIII CD133
Levels: CD133 EGFRvIII IL13Ra2
```

Now assume we wish to transform a numeric variable such as patients' age into a factor variable. There are different ways to do that in terms of number of levels we generate. In this instance, we wish to create levels such as "Elderly" and "MiddleAge," which denote patients above and below 60 years old, respectively. To do that, we create a fifth column as "AgeGroup":

```
> data$AgeGroup[data$Age<60]="MiddleAge"
> data$AgeGroup[data$Age>60]="Elderly"
> data
   Gender Age target.TAA Survival.mo.  AgeGroup
1       1  59    IL13Ra2            6 MiddleAge
2       1  63   EGFRvIII            5   Elderly
3       2  71    IL13Ra2           12   Elderly
4       1  67      CD133            4   Elderly
5       2  48   EGFRvIII           10 MiddleAge
6       1  78      CD133            6   Elderly
7       1  65    IL13Ra2            5   Elderly
8       2  65    IL13Ra2            7   Elderly
9       1  73   EGFRvIII            2   Elderly
10      2  78   EGFRvIII           NA   Elderly
11      1  56    IL13Ra2           14 MiddleAge
12      1  67      CD133            7   Elderly
13      2  69      CD133            9   Elderly
14      2  43    IL13Ra2            6 MiddleAge
15      2  58   EGFRvIII           NA MiddleAge
16      1  61      CD133            3   Elderly
17      1  60    IL13Ra2            5      <NA>
18      2  75   EGFRvIII           13   Elderly
19      2  66   EGFRvIII            7   Elderly
20      1  56      CD133           NA MiddleAge
```

The column created includes character variables:

```
> class(data[,5])
[1] "character"
```

However, we wish to convert their class to factor:

```
> data$AgeGroup=factor(data$AgeGroup, levels = c("Elderly","MiddleAge"))
> class(data[,5])
[1] "factor"
```

Matrices

Matrices, like vectors, store variables of the same class. However, unlike vectors, which are one-dimensional, matrices arrange their variables into a structure of fixed columns and rows; hence, they are two-dimensional.

As an example, we transform the vector D created by the function `seq()` into a matrix of four columns and five rows:

```
> D=seq(1,100, by=5)
> E=matrix(D, ncol=4, nrow=5, byrow =T)
> E
     [,1] [,2] [,3] [,4]
[1,]    1    6   11   16
[2,]   21   26   31   36
[3,]   41   46   51   56
[4,]   61   66   71   76
[5,]   81   86   91   96
```

In the matrix above, you can assign names to columns and rows:

```
> colnames(E)=c("Column1","Column2","Column3","Column4")
> rownames(E)=c("Row1","Row2","Row3", "Row4","Row5")
> E
     Column1 Column2 Column3 Column4
Row1       1       6      11      16
Row2      21      26      31      36
Row3      41      46      51      56
Row4      61      66      71      76
Row5      81      86      91      96
```

Data frames

Like matrixes, data frames are two-dimensional array-like arrangements of variables in which each column contains values of a variable, and each row can be considered a vector whose length is equal to the number of columns (variables). Many of the data sets that are commonly used in bioinformatics, such as gene expression data, etc., can be easily arranged into data frames.

As an example, imagine we have a data frame of infiltrating T lymphocytes into a certain tumor before and after vaccination in a sample of five tumors:

```
> samples=c("pt1","pt2","pt3","pt4","pt5")
> T_cells_before=c(23,54,25,17,43)
> T_cells_after=c(125,NA,143,178,92)
> G=data.frame(samples,T_cells_before,T_cells_after)
> G
  samples T_cells_before T_cells_after
1     pt1             23           125
2     pt2             54            NA
3     pt3             25           143
4     pt4             17           178
5     pt5             43            92
```

Unlike matrices, in data frames, columns are always assigned with names. All columns must be of same length, and the same holds true for rows as well. To create the data frame shown above, we combined the three vectors of samples, T_cells_before and T_cells_after. We can extend the columns and rows of data frames by using the functions `cbind()` and `rbind()`, which attach the vectors with a matching length to columns and rows of the existing data frame, respectively. An example is shown below:

```
> tumor_volume=c(24,19,22,17,25)
> New_G=cbind(G, tumor_volume)
> New_G
  samples T_cells_before T_cells_after tumor_volume
1     pt1             23           125           24
2     pt2             54            NA           19
3     pt3             25           143           22
4     pt4             17           178           17
5     pt5             43            92           25
```

Another method of adding this extra column to your data set would be defining the new column (as we did in the example of creating a factor variable of "AgeGroup" for glioblastoma [GBM] patients):

```
G$tumor_volume=c(24,19,22,17,25)
```

Importing data into R

You cannot always make your matrices or data frames by typing every detail in your source or console. Sometimes it is easier to prepare your spreadsheet data set in another software and then import it into your R session. R supports a variety of data formats, for example, comma/tab separated values (CSV/TSV), SPSS, Stata, and Excel to name a few. There are various ways of importing a data set from another file format to R. We mention below some of the options available for importing data from Excel into R as examples.

Importing data from the Environment window

In the introduction to the four windows of R, we mentioned that data can be imported into R from the Environment window. The package `readxl` is a prerequisite for importing data sets using this method. You can find the location of your data spreadsheet using the Browse menu next to the File/URL bar. At the bottom of the pop-up window, you can choose some features of how your data will be displayed.

Importing data using the `read.X()` command

Virtually all data formats can be imported into R by using the `read.X()` command, by substituting file format such as .csv, .delim, .table, _excel, .xlsx, etc. However, some of these commands, such as `read.xlsx()`, require installing packages such as `xlsx`. In the following examples, we overview some of these commands to open different data formats:

Example 1: `read.delim()`

Tab delimited is a common format for storing your data as text files. It is advisable to save your data in this format rather than CSV or spac-delimited, as many data include commas or space in their structure, which can be mistaken for commas and spaces that are set as separating arguments in CSV and space-delimited data sets. In tab delimited files, a separating argument is set to `"\t"`. In order to convert your data format from Excel file, SPSS, Stata, etc., into a tab-delimited format, go to File > Save As. In the pop-op window, you can choose the file format in which you wish to save your data. In order to save it as tab delimited, choose the Tab delimited option from the drop-down menu of the "Save as type" bar in order to import a tab delimited text file into R. Keep in mind that if you are converting data from Excel into tab delimited text, you need to create a separate text file for each sheet.

```
> Data -> read.delim("FileName.txt", header=T)
```

By setting the argument `header` as T (TRUE), you command R to set the first row of the data as row names.

Example 2: `read.csv()`

Importing data as CSV files, which are also saved as text files, is similar to importing data in a tab delimited format:

```
> Data -> read.csv("FileName.txt", header=T)
```

When importing data using the `read.X()` command, remember to set your working directory to the location where you have saved your file, unless you write the full address of your file location.

Example 3: `read.table()`

The `read.table()` function can import both tab- and space-delimited text files. This function creates a data frame from our text file. Much like the previous commands, this function, too, has a `header` argument that determines if the first row of the data set will be column names. Let us assume that we aim to import a tab-delimited text file named "GBM" from our working directory. In cases where our data set includes missing values (whose ways of handling will be discussed in detail in the next section), we must set the `fill` argument to TRUE.

```
> data=read.table("GBM.txt", header=TRUE, fill=TRUE)
> data
   Gender Age target.TAA Survival.mo.
1       1  59    IL13Ra2            6
2       1  63   EGFRvIII            5
3       2  71    IL13Ra2           12
4       1  67      CD133            4
5       2  48   EGFRvIII           10
6       1  78      CD133            6
7       1  65    IL13Ra2            5
8       2  65    IL13Ra2            7
9       1  73   EGFRvIII            2
10      2  78   EGFRvIII           NA
11      1  56    IL13Ra2           14
12      1  67      CD133            7
13      2  69      CD133            9
14      2  43    IL13Ra2            6
15      2  58   EGFRvIII           NA
16      1  61      CD133            3
17      1  60    IL13Ra2            5
18      2  75   EGFRvIII           13
19      2  66   EGFRvIII            7
20      1  56      CD133           NA
```

Example 4: `scan()`

The `scan()`function, unlike the previously mentioned methods, does not return a data frame of our data, but it creates a vector or a list. The type of data this function reads is defined by the `what` argument, which by default takes "numeric" values. However, if the argument `what` = or `what` = "character," it will read each value in the data set as a "character" value, irrespective of whether they are numbers or string characters. You are already familiar with the "GBM" data set. Let us import it into R using the `scan()` function:

```
> data=scan(file="GBM.txt", sep='\t', what="")
Read 84 items
> data
 [1] "Gender"    "Age "      "target.TAA" "Survival(mo)" "1"         "59"        "IL13R?2" "6"         "1"         "63"        "EGFRvIII"
[12] "5"         "2"         "71"        "IL13R?2"      "12"        "1"         "67"      "CD133"     "4"         "2"         "48"
[23] "EGFRvIII"  "10"        "1"         "78"           "CD133"     "6"         "1"       "65"        "IL13R?2"   "5"         "2"
[34] "65"        "IL13R?2"   "7"         "1"            "73"        "EGFRvIII"  "2"       "2"         "78"        "EGFRvIII"  ""
[45] "1"         "56"        "IL13R?2"   "14"           "1"         "67"        "CD133"   "7"         "2"         "69"        "CD133"
[56] "9"         "2"         "43"        "IL13R?2"      "6"         "2"         "58"      "EGFRvIII"  ""          "1"         "61"
[67] "CD133"     "3"         "1"         "60"           "IL13R?2"   "5"         "2"       "75"        "EGFRvIII"  "13"        "2"
[78] "66"        "EGFRvIII"  "7"         "1"            "56"        "CD133"     ""
```

You can see that the missing values appear as rather than NA, because the "scan" function simply reads every item and returns it inside a "." What is returned is a vector of character values:

```
> is.vector(data)
[1] TRUE
> class(data)
[1] "character"
```

If you do not set the `what` argument to "character" when reading data sets that include values other than numeric, you will receive an error, which will not be resolved until you set `what = character`. However, if your data set is made of entirely numeric values, the class of the values in the returned vector will be numeric as well, and the missing data will be shown as NA.

Copying data into clipboard

One easy way to import data into R is by copying data from spreadsheets into your clipboard (by pressing `ctrl + C` on Windows and `Command + C` in OSX). Shown below are the ways of import this data set into R:

In Windows:

```
> Data=read.table(file="clipboard",sep="\t",header=T)
```

In OSX:

```
> Data <- read.table(pipe("pbpaste"), sep="\t", header = TRUE)
```

Importing data from online sources

In order to import data sets from online sources, it is not necessary to save the data set in your device. There are many ways of importing data sets directly from an online source, some of which we will overview in this section:

1) read.csv() Function

```
> read.csv(url("http://some.where.net/data/example.csv"))
```

2) data.table Package

Another way of importing data from online sources is through using the `data.table` package. By using the `fread()` function, you can import data either from online sources or from a specific location on your device.

```
> data=fread("C:/Users/Immunoinformatics/Desktop/GBM.txt")

> data=fread("the url address")
```

Missing values

Let us create an imaginary data frame of GBM patient characteristics and their survival time. From the methods mentioned above for creating a data frame, it seems easier to create the table in an Excel file and then import data by copying them to clipboard. However, the choice of how to create the data frame is yours to make.

```
> data=read.table(file="clipboard",sep="\t",header=T)
> data
   Gender Age target.TAA Survival.mo.
1       1  59    IL13Ra2            6
2       1  63   EGFRvIII            5
3       2  71    IL13Ra2           12
4       1  67      CD133            4
5       2  48   EGFRvIII           10
6       1  78      CD133            6
7       1  65    IL13Ra2            5
8       2  65    IL13Ra2            7
9       1  73   EGFRvIII            2
10      2  78   EGFRvIII           NA
11      1  56    IL13Ra2           14
12      1  67      CD133            7
13      2  69      CD133            9
14      2  43    IL13Ra2            6
15      2  58   EGFRvIII           NA
16      1  61      CD133            3
17      1  60    IL13Ra2            5
18      2  75   EGFRvIII           13
19      2  66   EGFRvIII            7
20      1  56      CD133           NA
```

In the data set above, there are four features (variables) and 20 vectors displaying patient characteristics, including Gender, Age, Target TAA, and Survival (in months). However, due to various reasons such as loss of patient to follow-up, some vectors have missing values for the Survival feature. These missing values have been indicated by `NA`, which stands for "not available" in the data frame. Computations and mathematical operations on NA values will also result in NA values. For instance, we try to multiple by 3 all values of the Survival column in the data frame above. For this purpose, we extract the fourth column of the data set (`data[ ,4]` indicates any value that appears in the fourth column of the data set) and set it to the new value, which is three times their original value.

```
> data[,4]=data[,4]*3
> data
   Gender Age target.TAA Survival.mo.
1       1  59    IL13Ra2           18
2       1  63   EGFRvIII           15
3       2  71    IL13Ra2           36
4       1  67      CD133           12
5       2  48   EGFRvIII           30
6       1  78      CD133           18
7       1  65    IL13Ra2           15
8       2  65    IL13Ra2           21
9       1  73   EGFRvIII            6
10      2  78   EGFRvIII           NA
11      1  56    IL13Ra2           42
12      1  67      CD133           21
13      2  69      CD133           27
14      2  43    IL13Ra2           18
15      2  58   EGFRvIII           NA
16      1  61      CD133            9
17      1  60    IL13Ra2           15
18      2  75   EGFRvIII           39
19      2  66   EGFRvIII           21
20      1  56      CD133           NA
```

As was expected, all values but the missing ones are multiplied by 3. However, if we try to execute operations on a collection of values that include NA, the result will also be NA. For example, if we try to calculate the median or maximum value of the survival time for patients, we will get NA.

```
> median=median(data[,4])
> median
[1] NA
> max=max(data[,4])
> max
[1] NA
```

As performing many statistical measurements and calculating indices such as mean, median, mode, maximum, etc., requires all values to be available, we need to know whether our data set includes missing values. The `is.na()` function will help us find out if our data set includes missing values.

```
> is.na(data)
      Gender   Age target.TAA Survival.mo.
 [1,]  FALSE FALSE      FALSE        FALSE
 [2,]  FALSE FALSE      FALSE        FALSE
 [3,]  FALSE FALSE      FALSE        FALSE
 [4,]  FALSE FALSE      FALSE        FALSE
 [5,]  FALSE FALSE      FALSE        FALSE
 [6,]  FALSE FALSE      FALSE        FALSE
 [7,]  FALSE FALSE      FALSE        FALSE
 [8,]  FALSE FALSE      FALSE        FALSE
 [9,]  FALSE FALSE      FALSE        FALSE
[10,]  FALSE FALSE      FALSE         TRUE
[11,]  FALSE FALSE      FALSE        FALSE
[12,]  FALSE FALSE      FALSE        FALSE
[13,]  FALSE FALSE      FALSE        FALSE
[14,]  FALSE FALSE      FALSE        FALSE
[15,]  FALSE FALSE      FALSE         TRUE
[16,]  FALSE FALSE      FALSE        FALSE
[17,]  FALSE FALSE      FALSE        FALSE
[18,]  FALSE FALSE      FALSE        FALSE
[19,]  FALSE FALSE      FALSE        FALSE
[20,]  FALSE FALSE      FALSE         TRUE
```

If our data set is small, this function will be helpful. However, for larger data sets, we require other functions to indicate if there are missing values in our data set. For the sole purpose of knowing if there are missing values in a data set, the `any(is.na())` function is helpful. However, if we wish to know how many missing values we have throughout our data set, we can use the function `sum(is.na())`.

```
> any(is.na(data))
[1] TRUE

> sum(is.na(data))
[1] 3
```

In the data set "data," we know that we have three missing values. We can assign new values, for example, "3," "4," and "5," to these missing values:

```
> data[is.na(data)]=c(3,4,5)
> data
   Gender Age target.TAA Survival.mo.
1       1  59    IL13R?2            6
2       1  63   EGFRvIII            5
3       2  71    IL13R?2           12
4       1  67      CD133            4
5       2  48   EGFRvIII           10
6       1  78      CD133            6
7       1  65    IL13R?2            5
8       2  65    IL13R?2            7
9       1  73   EGFRvIII            2
10      2  78   EGFRvIII            3
11      1  56    IL13R?2           14
12      1  67      CD133            7
13      2  69      CD133            9
14      2  43    IL13R?2            6
15      2  58   EGFRvIII            4
16      1  61      CD133            3
17      1  60    IL13R?2            5
18      2  75   EGFRvIII           13
19      2  66   EGFRvIII            7
20      1  56      CD133            5
```

Another way of handling missing values is by omitting vectors that include missing values. In the example of GBM patients, this translates into removing all patients lost to follow-up from our calculations. One way is to remove rows that include NA values is by using the function `na.omit()`:

```
> data=na.omit(data)
> data
   Gender Age target.TAA Survival.mo.
1       1  59    IL13R?2            6
2       1  63   EGFRvIII            5
3       2  71    IL13R?2           12
4       1  67      CD133            4
5       2  48   EGFRvIII           10
6       1  78      CD133            6
7       1  65    IL13R?2            5
8       2  65    IL13R?2            7
9       1  73   EGFRvIII            2
11      1  56    IL13R?2           14
12      1  67      CD133            7
13      2  69      CD133            9
14      2  43    IL13R?2            6
16      1  61      CD133            3
17      1  60    IL13R?2            5
18      2  75   EGFRvIII           13
19      2  66   EGFRvIII            7
```

However, another way to handle missing values when we aim to perform statistical measurements and calculate indices is to set the `na.rm` argument as `TRUE`. In the example for indicating the median and maximum of the survival of GBM patients, we can calculate these indices without removing patients lost to follow-up in future calculations:

```
> median(data[ ,4], na.rm=TRUE)
[1] 6
> max(data[ ,4], na.rm=TRUE)
[1] 14
```

Organizing data

There are two main functions to organize your data in R: `sort()` and `order()`.

The `sort()` function takes a vector and sorts its values in either decreasing or increasing order, the default being increasing order (`decreasing = F`). Similar to the `max()` and `min()` functions, we must indicate how R should treat NA values; otherwise, R will remove (`na.last = NA`) these values by default when sorting the elements of the vector.

Let us take again the GBM data set to sort the values of the survival (the fourth column of the data frame):

```
> data=read.table("GBM.txt", header=TRUE)
> sort(data[,4])
 [1]  2  3  4  5  5  5  6  6  6  7  7  7  9 10 12 13 14
```

You can see that the values have been sorted in increasing order and the NA values have been omitted by default. In order to reverse the sorting method or change where in the sequence the NA values appear, we need to do the following:

```
> sort(data[,4], decreasing=T, na.last=T)
 [1] 14 13 12 10  9  7  7  7  6  6  6  5  5  5  4  3  2 NA NA NA
```

The `order()` function indicates the order of vector elements if they were to be sorted in increasing order:

```
> order(data[,4])
 [1]  9 16  4  2  7 17  1  6 14  8 12 19 13  5  3 18 11 10 15 20
```

Even though this function may not seem very useful per se, we can use it to sort the elements of one object based on another. For example, we may wish to sort the age of the GBM patients based on their survival to see if there is a meaningful relation between these two variables (however, investigating the relation between two variables can be easily performed using the `cor()` function, which surveys the correlation between two variables):

```
> Survival=data[,4]
> orderedSurvival=sort(data[,4])
> Age=data[,2]
> Age
 [1] 59 63 71 67 48 78 65 65 73 78 56 67 69 43 58 61 60 75 66 56
> orderedAge=Age[order(data[,4])]
> orderedAge
 [1] 73 61 67 63 65 60 59 78 43 65 67 66 69 48 71 75 56 78 58 56
```

In this new order, the values in each row of the Age and Survival columns correspond to one patient. However, patients lost to follow up have been placed at the end of the list as the NA values were placed in the corresponding positions of sorted survival.

Conditional statements in R

Conditional statements are one of the most important aspects of programming. They are based on logical and relational expressions and allow us to select a specific subset of our data that meet certain criteria and perform functions on them or exclude them from our computations, etc. Table 4.2 briefly reviews logical and relational operators.

Vectorized operators apply to all elements of a vector, while nonvectorized operators apply only to the first element of the vector.

There are different ways of indicating the conditions, but they all have one feature in common: they use a logical or relational expression as a filter to allow a function to be performed. We review some of the methods of conditional selection through conditional statements.

TABLE 4.2 Logical operators and their meaning in R.

Operator	Description
< or >	Less than or greater than
==	Equal to
!=	Not equal to
>=	Greater than or equal to
<=	Less than or equal to
| or ||	Or (vectorized vs nonvectorized)
& or &&	And (vectorized vs nonvectorized)

Indexing

In the previous sections, we learned about the square brackets [], which we used to select a row or a column of our data set. The square brackets are in fact indexing operators and they allow access to certain elements of the data. We can go further by selecting just columns and rows and select a subset of our data.

As an example, assume that we wish to evaluate the data of the patients aged between 60 and 70:

```
> datasubset=data[data$Age>60 & data$Age<70,]
> datasubset
   Gender Age target.TAA Survival.mo.
2       1  63   EGFRvIII            5
4       1  67      CD133            4
7       1  65    IL13R?2            5
8       2  65    IL13R?2            7
12      1  67      CD133            7
13      2  69      CD133            9
16      1  61      CD133            3
19      2  66   EGFRvIII            7
```

Note the "," inside the [], which indicates that we only want rows that meet the criteria. The `which()` function is another similar indexing method:

```
> datasubset=data[which(data$Age>60 & data$Age<70),]
> datasubset
   Gender Age target.TAA Survival.mo.
2       1  63   EGFRvIII            5
4       1  67      CD133            4
7       1  65    IL13R?2            5
8       2  65    IL13R?2            7
12      1  67      CD133            7
13      2  69      CD133            9
16      1  61      CD133            3
19      2  66   EGFRvIII            7
"If" Statements
```

The conditional statements are based on "if" statements. "If" the criterion is met, perform the function X; otherwise ("else"), perform the function Y. The basic conditional statements in R follow the frame below:

```
> if (logical condition) {
+   (command)
+   }
```

The "if" statement applies only to conditions of length 1, and if we try to apply them to a vector of length greater than 1, we get a warning.

As an example, in the GBM data set, we want to evaluate the overall survival (OS) of patients. Let us try the following conditional statement:

```
> if (survival>10){
+   print("Good OS")
+ }
Warning message:
In if (survival > 10) { :
  the condition has length > 1 and only the first element will be used
```

However, we can combine the "if" statements with loops or replace them with "`if else`" statements to resolve this limit. In the example above, if we try to investigate patient survival using "if" statements, we can create an index such as mean or median of survival to apply our logical statement to:

```
> survival=data[,4]
> Median_OS=median(survival, na.rm = TRUE)
> if (Median_OS<10){
+   print("Poor OS")
+ }
[1] "Poor OS"
```

Now that the logical statement holds true, R prints the character "Good OS." However, if the logical statement does not hold true, R will not perform any further action, as shown in the following example:

```
> if (Median_OS>10){
+   print("Good OS")
+ }
>
```

We can expand our conditional statement by creating more conditions so that R performs an action when either logical statements holds true:

```
> if (logical statement){
+   (command 1)

+ } else{
+   (command 2)
+ }
```

Therefore we can add another conditional statement to evaluate the survival of patients:

```
> if (Median_OS>10){
+   print("Good OS")
+ } else{
+   print("Poor OS")
+ }
[1] "Poor OS"
```

Since the median survival equals 6, the second logical statement is true. We can further expand the conditions:

```
> if (Median_OS>10){
+   print("Good OS")
+ } else{
+   if (Median_OS<5){
+     print("Poor OS")
+   }else{
+     print("Moderate OS")
+   }
+ }
[1] "Moderate OS"
```

Conditional statements with `ifelse`

It can be quite cumbersome to write conditional statements in the frame proposed above. There is an easier method (Fig. 4.2) of writing logical statements by using only one "if" statement and only one "else" statement.

Therefore the second-to-last example can be written as shown in the simple syntax below:

```
> ifelse(Median_OS>10, "Good OS", "Poor OS")
[1] "Poor OS"
```

In this chapter, we have briefly reviewed some of the basics of R programming. There is still more to fundamentals of programming in R, which will be discussed through the next chapters of the book.

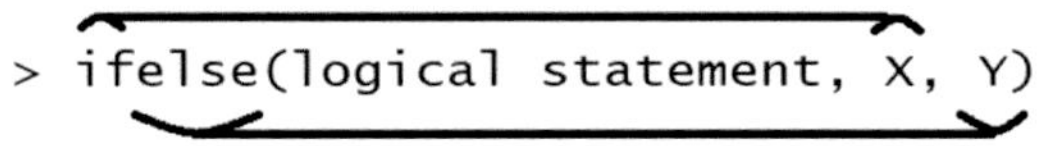

FIGURE 4.2 The `ifelse` logical statement. The `ifelse` function has three arguments: logical statement (test), command 1 (yes), which will be performed if the logical statement is true, and command 2 (no) if the statement is false.

SECTION III

ML algorithms and their applications

CHAPTER

5

Introduction to machine learning

What is machine learning?

Before we jump to the term machine learning (ML), it would be helpful to overview the concept of "learning." In essence, a myriad of results of searching for the meaning of "learning" are centered around the following concept: learning is the acquisition of brand-new knowledge as well as modifying knowledge and skills that have already been gained. This process, therefore, mandates observation and repetition until a new knowledge/skill is gained or modified. The learning process has been associated with animals and mankind throughout the history: they make observations of circumstances and the associated results, try to find the relation between these two, and try to apply this newfound knowledge to the same or similar upcoming situations.

Learning, therefore, can be regarded as a process of adaptation, which is observed not only at gross levels, being animal and human behavior, but also at much smaller levels, that is., at the cellular level. c. 1950, Donald Hebb observed that "when one cell repeatedly assists in firing another, the axon of the first cell develops synaptic knobs (or enlarges them if they already exist) in contact with the soma of the second cell." This can be regarded as an epitome of adaptation, which eventually led to the introduction of two intertwined terms: ML and artificial intelligence [1]. In the territory of these concepts, algorithms were developed that could remember previous inputs and results and could make decisions to improve the outcome in each iteration.

Hence, ML can be regarded as developing algorithms that enable computers to learn from iterative patterns in a way that they adapt their function parameters to improve to better reflect the events they are trained upon [2]. These events can be either structured data sets for some algorithms or unstructured data for some others, which rely on

DOI: https://doi.org/10.1016/B978-0-12-822400-7.00012-9

the algorithms to find undiscovered patterns in the data [3]. In this book, our focus will be on algorithms that use structured data sets to learn their recursive patterns and apply that knowledge in making predictions for unseen data.

Data structure

As mentioned earlier, there are two types of data that ML algorithms deal with: structured and nonstructured data. Structured data have labeled components, which makes it easier to understand the features of the data and visualize the entire data set. These data sets are the results of attempts to organize the data obtained from observations and experiments [3]. The data obtained directly from experiments are unstructured in the first place. Examples of unstructured data are manuscripts, images, websites, etc. Several of the databases discussed in Chapter 3 provide organized data sets that can be used for training ML algorithms.

In order to find the relationships between different components of a data set, we need to have a fair knowledge of the data structure. This is of utmost importance as the development of predictive models and clustering algorithms is not possible in the absence of knowledge regarding data structure.

Of the object types introduced in Chapter 4, data frames and matrices are the most suitable means to represent the data sets we face in bioinformatics: the big data. The high-throughput experiments performed today in studying organisms, which are the cornerstone of bioinformatics, generate petabytes of data. For instance, studying the expression of genes at the single-cell level with next-generation sequencing (scRNA-seq) generates data sets with tens of thousands of cases (rows in data frames and matrices), being the genes whose expression level in each cell is measured and thousands of variables (also referred to as attributes or features, columns of the table), being the cells whose gene expression levels have been examined. This data set can be considered as an example of the big data. Such data sets are too large in dimensions to be handled by traditional data processing methods.

Typically, structured data sets consist of independent variables (also known as features) and dependent variables (also known as response, outcome, or target variables) (Figs. 5.1 and 5.2).

How do machine learning algorithms treat big data?

Many algorithms have been developed to extract knowledge from both structured and nonstructured data. There are several ways of

Cases

Patient	Gender (Feature 1)	Age (Feature 2)	Target TAA (Feature 3)	Survival (months) (Feature 4 (Outcome))
1	Male	45	IL13Ra2	12
2	Male	63	EGFRvIII	8
3	Male	41	CD133	7
4	Female	53	EGFRvIII	15
5	Male	39	IL13Ra2	1
6	Female	50	IL13Ra2	19
7	Female	34	EGFRvIII	12
8	Male	61	CD133	9
9	Male	43	CD133	4
10	Female	70	IL13Ra2	10
11	Female	41	EGFRvIII	17
12	Male	23	IL13Ra2	4
13	Male	64	CD133	13
14	Female	39	CD133	1
15	Male	51	IL13Ra2	6
16	Male	50	EGFRvIII	7
17	Female	46	IL13Ra2	12
18	Female	40	IL13Ra2	9
19	Female	45	CD133	2
20	Male	63	EGFRvIII	14

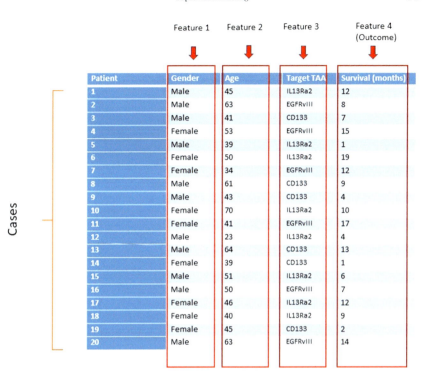

FIGURE 5.1 Structured data set to train a supervised learning algorithm. As the outcome variable is numerical, we implement regression algorithms to predict an output.

categorizing learning algorithms that have been developed thus far, and new algorithms are being developed constantly, affecting every aspect of life and science. We can broadly divide the already existing algorithms into supervised, unsupervised, semisupervised, and reinforcement learning algorithms. Discussion of each of these algorithms is beyond the scope of this book as we only focus on supervised learning algorithms. The choice between these types of learning depends mostly on the structure (or lack of structure) of the data and the purpose of using ML algorithms.

Supervised learning

Many of the practical ML algorithms deal with structured data and hence are supervised learning algorithms. In supervised learning, we "feed" our model with a well-structured data set that consists of labeled variables and a specific outcome (Figs. 5.1 and 5.2). This data set is called a training data set, as our model takes instances from this data

Cases

Patient	Gender (Feature 1)	Age (Feature 2)	Target TAA (Feature 3)	Survival (Feature 4 (Outcome))
1	Male	45	IL13Ra2	Good
2	Male	63	EGFRvIII	Poor
3	Male	41	CD133	Poor
4	Female	53	EGFRvIII	Good
5	Male	39	IL13Ra2	Poor
6	Female	50	IL13Ra2	Good
7	Female	34	EGFRvIII	Good
8	Male	61	CD133	Poor
9	Male	43	CD133	Poor
10	Female	70	IL13Ra2	Poor
11	Female	41	EGFRvIII	Good
12	Male	23	IL13Ra2	Poor
13	Male	64	CD133	Good
14	Female	39	CD133	Poor
15	Male	51	IL13Ra2	Poor
16	Male	50	EGFRvIII	Poor
17	Female	46	IL13Ra2	Good
18	Female	40	IL13Ra2	Poor
19	Female	45	CD133	Poor
20	Male	63	EGFRvIII	Good

FIGURE 5.2 Structured data set to train a supervised learning algorithm. As the outcome variable is categorical, we implement classification algorithms to predict an output.

set to infer a relationship between the variables and the outcome. Therefore, the purpose of this model is to make predictions based on the inferred relationship between the variables. Based on the type of the outcome, whether it is a number (numerical or continuous variable) or a factor (categorical or discrete variable), the algorithms that we implement to make predictions are regression or classification algorithms, respectively. Therefore, to make predictions on the survival of patients presented in Fig. 5.1, we must use a regression algorithm. Regression algorithms use various functions to find the relationship between variables and the numeric output. Once trained using a structured data set, they can find numeric outcomes for new observations given that the variables based on which the algorithm-trained models are provided for these observations.

However, if our response variable (output) is a categorical or ordinal variable, classification algorithms will be used to decipher the relationship between independent and dependent variables. As an example, if we categorized patients in Fig. 5.1 based on their survival into those with a good prognosis (survival $>$ 10 months) or a poor prognosis (survival $\leq$ 10 months) as outlined in Fig. 5.2, we must implement classification algorithms.

The rest of the chapters in this book are primarily concerned with different regression and classification algorithms, and how to make the choice of which algorithm to choose.

Principles of training the model

The main purpose of implementing ML algorithms is to predict the outcomes of a new observation. This is what can help us inform a 32-year-old female patient with glioblastoma expressing EGFRvIII about the prognosis of her disease. For this, we have to rely on the generalizability of the model we trained with either of the data sets presented in Figs. 5.1 or 5.2. In order to generalize, our model tries to create a polynomial equation based on the instances in the data set. Each ML algorithm uses different functions, and using the information gained from the data set, it adopts the parameters of the function to best reflect the data set [3]. This way, for the instance of most algorithms, when we want to know the outcome for a new patient, we can simply find the answer to the functions used by the algorithms.

In order to "train" our model, we provide instances to the functions used by the algorithms so that the parameters of these functions are adjusted. It is evident that the more observations are presented to the model, the better adjustment of model parameters will be, and the more accurate its predictions will be when faced with a new observation. In order to make sure that the predictions of the model are reliable, we need to test its predictions with unseen data. In order to do so, we test the model with observations in the data set it was trained upon. If the model performs well in making predictions for these testing data, it can be used for making an accurate prediction on similar observations. Therefore, in practice, when training ML models, we divide our data sets into two to three subsets, based on the size of the data set. If our data set is large enough, we divide the instances of the data set into three groups: training, validation, and testing. The proportions based on which we classify our data set into these three categories are rather arbitrary. However, if our data set is large enough, a good proportion would be about 2:1:1, and if we do not have a rather large data set, dividing them as 3:1:1 would be good practice. However, in practice, data sets are mostly divided into training and testing subsets. The purpose of this division is to test our model for its generalizability, accuracy, and the possibility of overfitting. These concepts will be discussed throughout the book. Furthermore, it is important to know that this categorization, on its own, will not be enough to guarantee a good model in terms of accuracy and generalizability. We need to ensure that the instances in our data set are randomly attributed to these three groups so that the order of what we present to our model does not affect its function. For instance, if we feed our model only with instances of male glioblastoma patients expressing EGFRvIII, our model will be naïve when faced with an instance of a female glioblastoma patient expressing CD133.

There are some other methods to train a model, especially if the data set is really small, without necessarily dividing our data set into three groups: training, validation, and testing. Of these methods, *multifold cross validation* and *leave-one-out* can be named [4]. In these methods, we make use of all instances in our data set to train the model. For example, in K-fold cross-validation, we randomly divide our data set into K subsets, and at each iteration, we leave one of these K subsets aside for validation purposes and train the model with the $K-1$ subsets. We repeat the training process until all K subsets are used to train the model. Each training fold will result in the creation of a separate model, and the general model will be created by K-fold cross validation of the average of all K models created on each of the K subsets.

Once we have decided on how to divide our data into training and testing subsets, we must move forward to building the model itself. As an example, we aim to build a regression model on the survival of patients based on the data in hand regarding the number of tumor-infiltrating lymphocytes. The data regarding patient survival and the number of tumor-infiltrating lymphocytes are depicted in Fig. 5.3. A glance at the dots clearly indicates that as the number of tumor-infiltrating lymphocytes increases, the patient will have a better prognosis. But if we are interested in a more accurate estimation on the prognosis of the patients based on the number of tumor-infiltrating lymphocytes, we need to create a model representing the relationship between these two variables. Different models will try different equations to see which one represents this relationship better. Let us consider different equations for this purpose, starting from the simplest form, that is., first-degree polynomial that follows a linear trend

$$\text{Model A:} \quad y = ax + c \tag{5.1}$$

where y is the survival of the patient, a is the coefficient (slope) of the line, x is the number of tumor-infiltrating lymphocytes, and c is the y-intercept. Fig. 5.4 shows the schematic line representing Model A.

As can be deduced, Model A is not the best representative of the relationship between patient survival and the number of tumor-infiltrating lymphocytes. Therefore, we try a more complicated model

$$\text{Model B:} \quad y = ax^2 + bx + c \tag{5.2}$$

This second-degree polynomial results in a curve, as shown in Fig. 5.5.

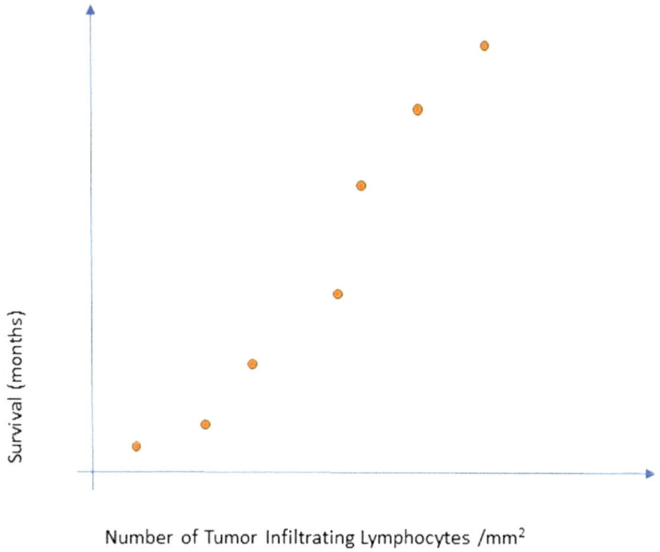

FIGURE 5.3 Dot plot of patients' survival-based and number of tumor-infiltrating lymphocytes.

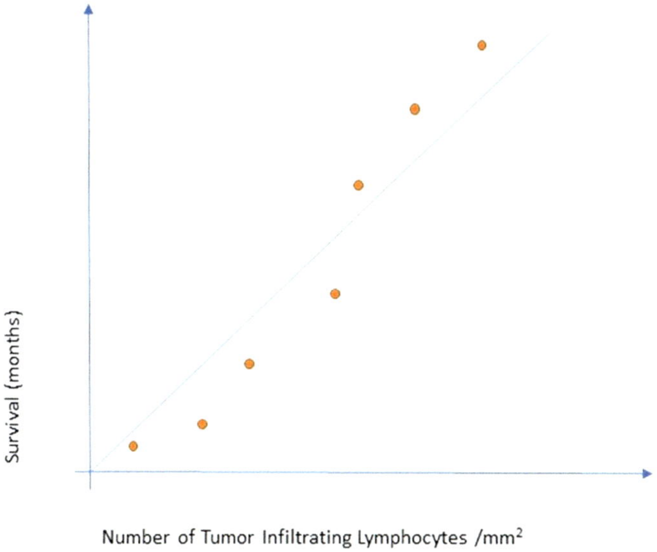

FIGURE 5.4 The line represents a first-degree polynomial model attempting to generalize the relationship between patients' survival and the number of tumor-infiltrating lymphocytes.

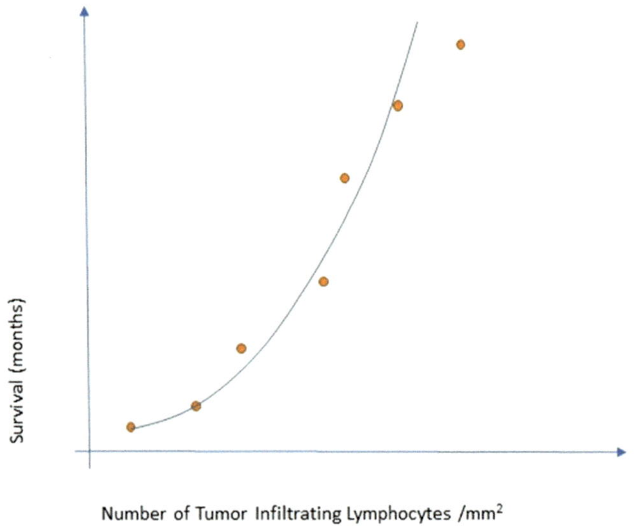

FIGURE 5.5 The curve represents a second-degree polynomial model attempting to generalize the relationship between patients' survival and the number of tumor-infiltrating lymphocytes.

In these regression algorithms, the purpose is to find the line or the curve that passes as close as possible to all the points in the dot plot. For this purpose, the algorithms try different parameters for the general function of the model, as shown in Eqs. 5.1 and 5.2, to find the one that best describes the data set, based on the instances that we feed our model. In more complicated algorithms, attempts are made to find decision boundaries or assign weights to features, in such a way that predictions are as close as possible to the actual values of observations.

A similar method applies to classification algorithms as well. The aim of classification models is to generate decision boundaries or appropriate weights for features that can effectively classify the instances within a data set. These decision boundaries can be lines, curves, or hyperplanes based on the distribution of the instances within the vector space as well as the number of the features we choose to build our model upon, which determines the dimensionality of our model. This brings us to one of the most important aspects of ML: feature selection.

Feature selection

Once making a model, there are many parameters that we must decide beforehand based on the data we have in hand and our purposes. As mentioned earlier, the nature of the data generated in biological studies is that of the big data. This means that there are thousands of columns and rows (features and instances, respectively) in the data frames and matrices representing them.

As a rule of thumb, we need about 10 instances for each feature that we include in building our model so that different patterns can be iterated enough for our model to learn the association between features and outcomes. There are, however, more complicated ways of finding the appropriate size of the data set for making predictive models [5]. Given the fact that we cannot change the number of our instances in many cases once the experiment and data collection phase is done, we need to manipulate the number of features based on which we build our model. There are various methods to reduce the number of features in our model, which are generally referred to as feature selection methods. In addition, there are other ways of dealing with a large number of features in data sets, which is generally termed dimensionality reduction [6].

It is important to choose distinguishing features to build our model because choosing features mutual among the majority of instances within a data set only increases the dimensionality of our model, which, in turn, increases the time and the size of the data set our model requires to perform the predictions, without actually helping with distinguishing one instance from another. An example of such features is housekeeping genes that are expressed in high levels in different cell types. Many of the feature selection methods automatically factor in such similarities when choosing features for building models.

The various methods of feature selection can be broadly divided into three categories: wrapper methods, filter methods, and embedded methods.

Wrapper methods are the best methods for feature selection; however, they require high levels of computation, which is costly and time-consuming. There are two main methods in this category: recursive feature elimination and forward feature selection. In the former, our primary model is built based on all the features, and at this stage, a certain weight is attributed to each feature. At each iteration, the feature with the least weight is removed. As long as the model improves with the elimination of features, this process continues. In forward feature selection, the reverse of recursive feature elimination is performed. Once weights have been attributed to each feature following building the model based on all features, we can factor in features with the most weights. This process will continue as long as the model improves during cross validation [7].

In filter methods, different statistical methods are used to assign different coefficients to the features. These coefficients are indicative of the correlation between the outcome and each feature. Some of the statistical methods for computing these coefficients include Pearson's correlation, analysis of variance (ANOVA), chi-square, linear discriminant analysis, and quadratic discriminant analysis. The two latter are also used for classification purposes in addition to dimension reduction [8].

Finally, embedded methods integrate the feature selection and learning process. This is more efficient in terms of calculation time. Decision trees are good examples of performing feature selection as part of training the model. At each iteration of the learning process, the algorithm decides which features are important to keep and which ones can be removed from constructing the model. Some of the most implemented of these methods are L1 (Lasso), L2 (Ridge), and L1/L2 regularizations (elastic nets). In L1 regularization, the coefficients of some parameters (features) shrink to zero, which will lead to their elimination from the final predictive model. Even though L2 regularization also shrinks the coefficients based on their importance, as it never shrinks them to zero, the L1 regularization is more efficient for the elimination of unpredictive features [9].

There are several methods of dimensionality reduction, especially in the field of bioinformatics [10]. One of the most well-known methods of dimensionality reduction is principal component analysis (PCA), which is briefly discussed in this chapter.

Principal component analysis

As mentioned before, the dimensionality of a predictive model equals the number of features included in building that model. In a coordinate system, this translates to assigning an axis to each variable. Our aim by performing PCA is to rotate the coordinate of the data in such a way that each axis reflects as much variance of the data as possible. Therefore, in PCA, the number of the components equals the number of the features included in building the data. It is important to keep in mind that PCA must be implemented only on continuous data. The first component is the one that reflects the highest levels of data variance. In a relatively small data set, the first few components explain most of the data variability [10].

Even though PCA provides us with fewer components to build our model upon, it is harder to interpret. We build our model upon components that mirror variability of our features, not the features themselves. In order to better understand the struggles with the interpretation of a model based on PCA, consider the following example:

We aim to model the survival of glioblastoma patients based on the following imaginary data on their treatment regimens:

```
> data
   age sex metastasis stage chemotherapy surgery radiotherapy  OS
1   69   1          0     1            0       2            0 108
2   18   2          0     1            0       2            0 258
3   13   1          0     1            0       2            0 231
4   30   1          0     2            0       1            1  73
5   36   1          0     2            0       1            1  24
6   12   2          0     3            1       1            1  14
7   17   1          0     3            1       0            1  12
8   14   1          0     3            1       0            1 307
9   15   2          0     3            1       0            0  62
10  32   1          0     3            1       0            1 124
11  12   2          0     3            1       2            0  97
12  17   1          1     4            1       0            0   9
13  14   1          1     4            1       0            1  24
14  19   1          1     4            1       1            1  17
15  12   1          1     4            1       0            1  12
16  17   2          1     4            1       0            1  16
17  18   1          1     4            1       0            1  60
18  20   2          1     4            1       0            1  15
19  15   1          1     4            1       1            0  36
20  21   2          1     4            1       1            1  33
21  25   2          1     4            1       1            0  18
22  19   1          1     4            1       1            0  40
23  15   1          1     4            1       2            0  68
24  17   2          1     4            2       0            0  44
25  14   2          1     4            2       0            1 125
26  12   1          1     4            2       2            0  39
27  23   2          1     4            2       2            1 104
```

In order to find the principal components, we use the function `prcomp()`. As we aim to find the importance of each feature in the predictive model, we leave the outcome (survival) column out of calculations:

```
> pca=prcomp(data[,-8])
> pca
Standard deviations (1, .., p=7):
[1] 11.5672065  1.1348245  0.7790042  0.5070653  0.4176619  0.3236703
0.1984813

Rotation (n x k) = (7 x 7):
                      PC1         PC2         PC3         PC4          PC5          PC6          PC7
age          -0.998527976  0.05237820  0.01027048  0.00689082 -0.003697152  0.003214299  0.004630153
sex           0.008219275  0.02739481  0.11325883  0.92243452 -0.045075550 -0.361355538  0.053472654
metastasis    0.013282914  0.31718838  0.27277224 -0.17512536 -0.016605942 -0.449010309 -0.769581378
stage         0.043511154  0.75459070  0.30457440 -0.14642004  0.057427055 -0.147667684  0.537951347
chemotherapy  0.023150589  0.33064265  0.25353854  0.29112455 -0.008861959  0.803680353 -0.308421061
surgery      -0.016340467 -0.43878723  0.79281328 -0.07005176  0.403045882  0.001478990  0.106256460
radiotherapy  0.001306660  0.15694478 -0.35645758  0.08543181  0.912061612 -0.009567833 -0.095174054

> class(pca)
[1] "prcomp"
```

As expected, the number of principal components equals the number of features. As noted, in each principal component, a number is attributed to each feature, which indicates the correlation of each principal component with that feature. These correlation coefficients range between -1 and 1. For example, the correlation coefficient between age and PC1 is approximately -0.998. This indicates a negative correlation between age and PC1, meaning as the age increases, PC1 decreases. But how do we decide which principal components should we choose?

As mentioned earlier, the first principal is the one that explains the highest level of variability within features, and the first few components explain the majority of variability. In order to find the variability explained by each component, we use the function `summary()`.

```
> summary(pca)
Importance of components:
                           PC1     PC2     PC3     PC4     PC5     PC6     PC7
Standard deviation     11.5672 1.13482 0.77900 0.50707 0.41766 0.32367 0.19848
Proportion of Variance  0.9819 0.00945 0.00445 0.00189 0.00128 0.00077 0.00029
Cumulative Proportion   0.9819 0.99132 0.99578 0.99766 0.99894 0.99971 1.00000
```

In the table above, the line "Proportion of variance" indicates how much of the variability of features is explained by each component. As can be noted, the principal components appear in order of importance in terms of explaining data variability. The first two components are often used to build the model as they explain the majority of data variability. The importance of each component in each of these components can be understood either from calling the "prcomp" (in the example above named "pca") or from the biplot of the PCA (Fig. 5.6):

```
> biplot(pca)
```

As can be seen in Fig. 5.6, it is hard to appreciate the details of this biplot. We can make the plot more informative by making some changes to how it is presented (Fig. 5.7):

```
> biplot(pca, xlim=c(-0.2, 0.2), ylim=c(-0.2, 0.2), expand=10)
```

The biplots indicate that "age" and "stage" are the most important features of the PC1 and PC2, respectively.

Using principal components in order to reduce the dimensionality of our model reduces training time and possibility of overfitting, in addition to increasing the accuracy or reliability of our model, which is the most important property of a model.

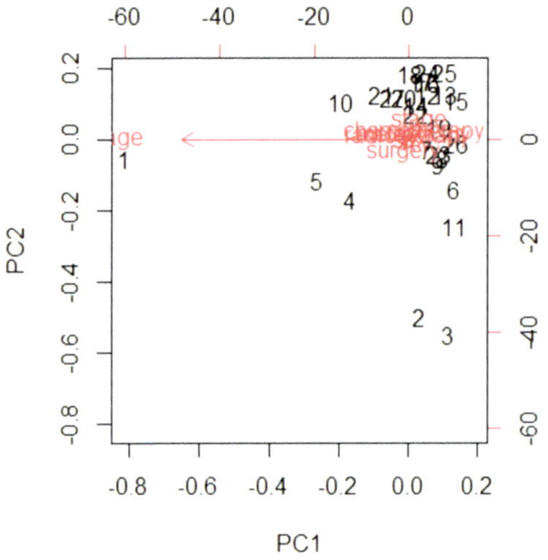

FIGURE 5.6 Biplot of the PCA.

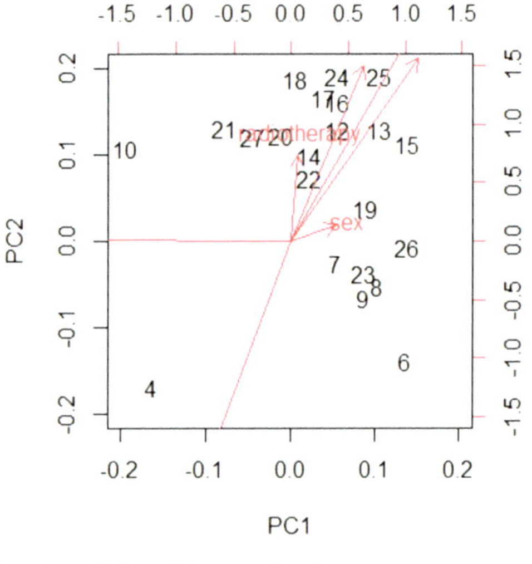

FIGURE 5.7 Biplot of the PCA with more details.

Accuracy

There are various ways of determining how well a classification model performs: accuracy, recall, and precision are some of these methods. However, what we focus on throughout the book to compare various classification models is the accuracy of the model.

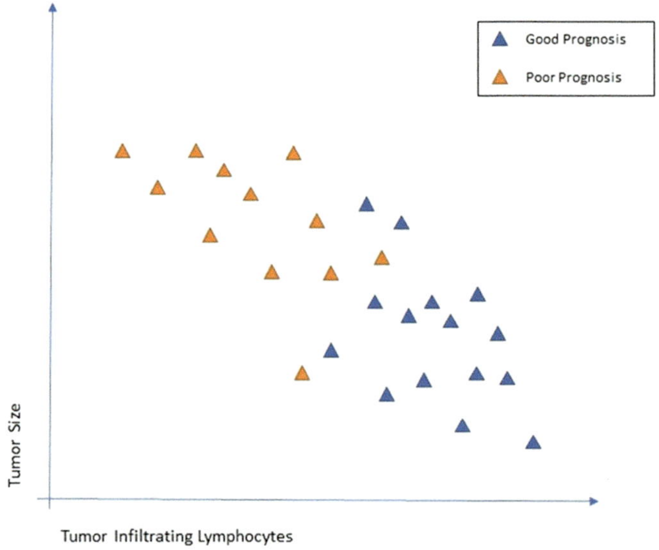

FIGURE 5.8 Dot plot of patients based on their tumor size and tumor-infiltrating lymphocytes.

Accuracy is the ability of a classification model to correctly classify observations. Consider a data set of patients' prognosis as of good prognosis and poor prognosis, their tumor size, and number of tumor-infiltrating lymphocytes (Fig. 5.8). We aim to find a model that can classify patients into those with good prognosis and poor prognosis based on their tumor size and number of tumor-infiltrating lymphocytes. The purpose of this model is to classify patients into the aforementioned groups as correctly as possible, meaning that all data points representative of patients with good prognosis are placed on one side of the decision boundary, whereas all patients with poor prognosis are placed on the other side of the decision boundary. Figs. 5.9 and 5.10 show the schematic representation of two models for this purpose. How do we know which model is better? That is a question of the accuracy of the model and its generalizability.

One simple way of determining the accuracy of a model is the confusion matrix, which is a matrix of actual classes of observations vs predicted classes. This confusion matrix allows us to understand how many data sets have been correctly classified. In order to find the accuracy of a model, we need to divide the number of correctly classified observations by the total number of observations. This concept is elaborated with more details in future chapters.

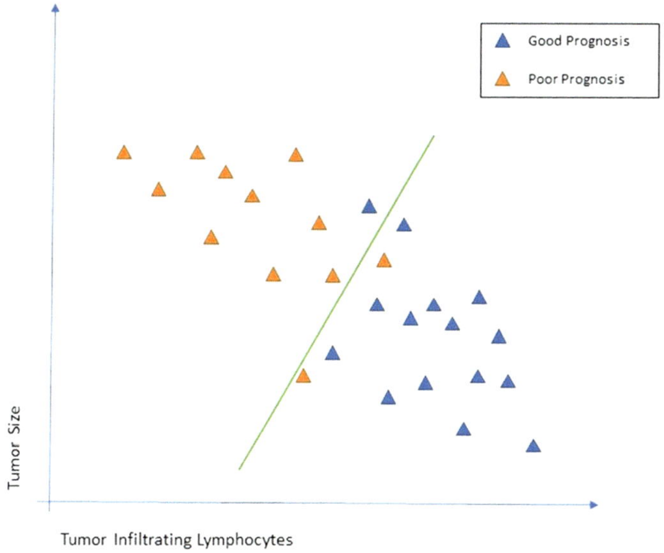

FIGURE 5.9 A classification model generating a simple decision boundary (green line). This model has misclassified a total of three instances (two patients with poor prognosis are classified as good prognosis, and one patient with good prognosis is classified as poor prognosis).

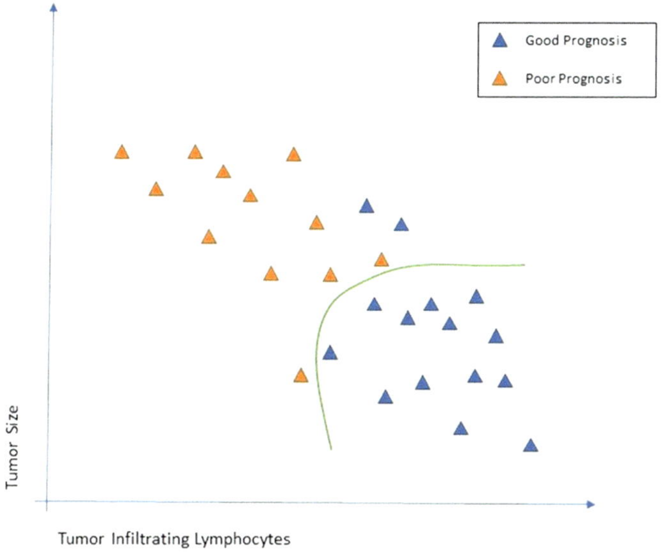

FIGURE 5.10 A relatively complicated classification model. This model has misclassified a total of two instances.

Performance metrics of regression models

Similar to classification models, for regression models, we need indices of the model's performance to have an estimate of how reliable predictions of our model are and to compare the performance of different models with one another. Unlike classification models, we do not choose a label for each observation, and therefore, we cannot use a hit-or miss-based method, such as a confusion matrix, to find how good the predictions of our model are. In order for regression models to have reliable predictions, their predicted values must be as close as possible to the observations' actual values. There are different methods to evaluate this closeness of predictions to actual values; root mean squared error (RMSE), R squared and adjusted R squared, and Akaike's information criteria are a few of these methods. In this book, we focus on RMSE for comparison of our regression models, which will be discussed in future chapters.

Generalizability of models

We mentioned that in order to train our models, we use a subset of the data we have and reserve the rest of the observations in the data set for validation and testing our model. The reason behind this is to determine how generalizable predictions of our model are. In other words, how well our data can perform when faced with previously unseen data.

If we use all the observations in the data set to train our model, the performance of our model will increase. This is due to the fact that the proportion of observations to features increases, and for each feature, there are more observations available, and the probability of recursive patterns increases. If we test our model using the same observations it was trained upon, its performance will be remarkable. However, such an index is not a good judge of the model's performance, as our model is "memorizing" events to some extent. Therefore, we need to test our model's performance using the testing subset of data. If a model's performance in making predictions for training subset is remarkably better than its performance in predicting a testing subset, our model is "overfitting" on the training data and its predictions are not reliable.

In addition to the data upon which a model is trained, there are other factors that can lead to overfitting and generalizability of the model. The algorithms and parameters used to train the model play a major role in its generalizability, as some of the ML algorithms are more prone to overfitting than others. These concepts will be reviewed in future chapters.

In this chapter, we briefly introduced some of the basic concepts in ML. In the rest of the chapters, we use these concepts to create regression and classification models using examples and real-world data sets.

References

[1] J.L. Krichmar, J.L. Olds, J.V. Sanchez-Andres, H. Tang, Editorial: explainable artificial intelligence and neuroscience: cross-disciplinary perspectives, Frontiers in Neurorobotics 15 (2021) 731733. Available from: https://doi.org/10.3389/fnbot.2021.731733.

[2] R.Y. Choi, A.S. Coyner, J. Kalpathy-Cramer, M.F. Chiang, J.P. Campbell, Introduction to machine learning, neural networks, and deep learning, Translational Vision Science & Technology 9 (2) (2020) 14. Available from: https://doi.org/10.1167/tvst.9.2.14.

[3] D. Zhang, C. Yin, J. Zeng, X. Yuan, P. Zhang, Combining structured and unstructured data for predictive models: a deep learning approach, BMC Medical Informatics and Decision Making 20 (1) (2020) 280. Available from: https://doi.org/10.1186/s12911-020-01297-6.

[4] I. Tougui, A. Jilbab, J.E. Mhamdi, Impact of the choice of cross-validation techniques on the results of machine learning-based diagnostic applications, Healthcare Informatics Research 27 (3) (2021) 189–199. Available from: https://doi.org/10.4258/hir.2021.27.3.189.

[5] I. Balki, A. Amirabadi, J. Levman, A.L. Martel, Z. Emersic, B. Meden, et al., Sample-size determination methodologies for machine learning in medical imaging research: a systematic review, Canadian Association of Radiologists journal = Journal l'Association canadienne des radiologistes 70 (4) (2019) 344–353. Available from: https://doi.org/10.1016/j.carj.2019.06.002.

[6] B. Mwangi, T.S. Tian, J.C. Soares, A review of feature reduction techniques in neuroimaging, Neuroinformatics 12 (2) (2014) 229–244. Available from: https://doi.org/10.1007/s12021-013-9204-3.

[7] Y. Mao, Y. Yang, A wrapper feature subset selection method based on randomized search and multilayer structure, BioMed Research International 2019 (2019) 9864213. Available from: https://doi.org/10.1155/2019/9864213.

[8] A. Bommert, T. Welchowski, M. Schmid, J. Rahnenführer, Benchmark of filter methods for feature selection in high-dimensional gene expression survival data, Briefings in Bioinformatics, bbab354. Advance Online Publication (2021). Available from: https://doi.org/10.1093/bib/bbab354.

[9] A.C. Haury, P. Gestraud, J.P. Vert, The influence of feature selection methods on accuracy, stability and interpretability of molecular signatures, PLoS One 6 (12) (2011) e28210. Available from: https://doi.org/10.1371/journal.pone.0028210.

[10] C. Meng, O.A. Zeleznik, G.G. Thallinger, B. Kuster, A.M. Gholami, A.C. Culhane, Dimension reduction techniques for the integrative analysis of multi-omics data, Briefings in Bioinformatics 17 (4) (2016) 628–641. Available from: https://doi.org/10.1093/bib/bbv108.

CHAPTER

6

Naïve Bayes' classifiers in R

An introduction to Bayes' theorem

As this chapter is the first chapter of our hands-on machine learning experience in R, we will learn about one of the most useful algorithms in machine learning known as Bayes' classification algorithm. This algorithm is a supervised learning algorithm that, while being simple, can efficiently classify data points into different classes. There are different types of Bayes' classifiers all of which are based on Bayes' theorem; however, Bayes' theorem is used in many other classification algorithms as well. Bayes' theorem was established in the 18th century by an English statistician, Thomas Bayes. As this theorem is the basis of many classification algorithms, it is important to understand Bayes' theorem.

Bayes' theorem helps us with finding the probability of an event given a set of prior knowledge. The equation to calculate such probability is [1]:

$$P(A|B) = \frac{P(B|A)P(A)}{P(B)}, \tag{6.1}$$

where $P(A|B)$, also known as *posterior probability*, is the probability that event A occurs given that the condition B is true and $P(B|A)$ is the probability that the condition B is true given that the event A occurs, which is also known as "likelihood." $P(A)$, or *class prior probability of A*, and $P(B)$, or *predictor prior probability*, are the probability of event A and condition B being true, respectively, independent of other circumstances.

The most well-known of classifiers based on Bayes' theorem is Naïve Bayes' classifier. The algorithm assumes that the independent variables are independent, hence called Naïve. Even though in biological data this assumption does not always hold true, Naïve Bayes' classifier is still used for many classification purposes as it is faster

DOI: https://doi.org/10.1016/B978-0-12-822400-7.00010-5

compared to other classification algorithms and requires less computer memory [2].

Since the main assumption of Naïve Bayes' is independence of variables, not every data can be properly classified using this algorithm. As can be seen in Eq. (6.1), in order to calculate the likelihood of different conditions, we need to calculate their ratios (explained later). Therefore, if our variables are continuous, this method is not going to be as efficient as for the classification of a data set with categorical variables [3]. Even though we can recode the numeric variables to categorical variables based on some classification methods such as quartiles, this will not accurately reflect the effects of the numerical variables on the dependent variable. However, there are more complex methods to employ Naïve Bayes' for classification based on continuous variables [4,5], one way to avoid complex models is to reserve Naïve Bayes' for the classification of a data set composed of only categorical independent variables. However, if we choose to use Naïve Bayes' for data sets with numeric variables, the probabilities of any value will be determined based on the distribution of the data points along with other factors such as mean value for that variables, which will be further discussed in Chapter 16 through practice examples.

In this chapter, in order to understand the effect of data set's structure on the performance of classification models, we will use two data sets. One of these data sets, composed of categorical and numeric covariates, will be used to develop other classification models in forthcoming chapters and compare the performance of different algorithms for the same data set. The other data set is composed of only categorical covariates and includes patients' histopathologic findings, chemotherapy regimen, and their survival (Table 6.1). We want to create a model to predict patients' survival based on these characteristics. In practice, the dimension of the data is several times larger, which could require feature selection; however, for demonstrative purposes, we start by explaining Bayes' theorem with regard to this data set and try to create a classification model. Expectedly, our classification model will not be as good as a classification model created using a larger data set composed of several observations. However, for our learning purposes, we use a rather small data set, and discuss the challenges that can arise from using a small data set to train Naïve Bayes' classifier.

Based on the data shown in Table 6.1, let us calculate the probability of a patient having long survival if they have received regimen C, and in their tumor microenvironment, they have increased levels of matrix metalloproteinases (MMPs) and an M2 tumor associated macrophage (TAM). Let us first calculate the prior probabilities of classes and predictors:

TABLE 6.1 Example data set of patients' response to chemotherapy.

Regimen	TAM	Increased MMP	Survival
A	M1	Yes	Intermediate
C	M1	No	Long
A	M2	Yes	Short
B	M1	Yes	Long
B	M1	No	Long
B	M2	No	Long
C	M1	No	Long
A	M2	Yes	Short
C	M2	No	Intermediate
A	M2	Yes	Short
B	M1	Yes	Intermediate
A	M2	No	Intermediate
C	M1	Yes	Intermediate
A	M1	No	Long
C	M1	No	Long
B	M1	No	Long
B	M2	No	Intermediate
B	M2	Yes	Short
C	M1	No	Long
C	M1	Yes	Intermediate
A	M1	Yes	Intermediate
A	M2	No	Intermediate
B	M1	No	Long
A	M1	No	Long
C	M2	Yes	Short
A	M1	No	Long
B	M1	No	Long
A	M2	Yes	Short
A	M2	No	Intermediate
C	M1	Yes	Intermediate

MMP, Matrix metalloproteinase; *TAM*, tumor associated macrophage.

$$prior\ probability\ of\ regimen\ A = \frac{12}{30} \times 100 = 40\%$$

$$prior\ probability\ of\ regimen\ B = \frac{9}{30} \times 100 = 30\%$$

$$prior\ probability\ of\ regimen\ C = \frac{9}{30} \times 100 = 30\%$$

$$prior\ probability\ of\ M1 = \frac{18}{30} \times 100 = 60\%$$

$$prior\ probability\ of\ M2 = \frac{12}{30} \times 100 = 40\%$$

$$prior\ probability\ of\ increased\ MMP = \frac{13}{30} \times 100 \cong 43\%$$

$$prior\ probability\ of\ normal\ MMP = \frac{17}{30} \times 100 \cong 67\%$$

$$prior\ probability\ of\ long\ survival = \frac{13}{30} \times 100 \cong 43\%$$

$$prior\ probability\ of\ intermediate\ survival = \frac{11}{30} \times 100 \cong 37\%$$

$$prior\ probability\ of\ short\ survival = \frac{6}{30} \times 100 = 20\%$$

To calculate the probability of long survival in a patient with increased MMPs and M2 TAM after chemotherapy with regimen C, we need to calculate

$$P(long\ survival|M2,\ increased\ MMP,\ regimen\ C)$$

$$= \frac{P(M2|long)\ P(increased\ MMP|long)\ P(regimen\ C|long)\ P(long)}{P(M2)\ P(increased\ MMP)\ P(regimen\ C)}$$

As an example, the probability $P(increased\ MMP|,long)$ is 1/13, meaning that out of 13 patients with long survival, one has increased MMP levels.

Hands-on Naïve Bayes' in R

There are several R packages developed to train Naïve Bayes classifiers in R. Even though using these packages is easy, developing classification models with Naïve Bayes' algorithm in R can be frustrating to some extent. There can be several error and warning messages, some of which inherent to the nature of the functions in some of the packages used for developing Naïve Bayes' classifiers. In this chapter, we will discuss how to resolve some of the issues that may arise while training Naïve Bayes' classifiers.

The first set of data we will use to train our classifier is the data set presented in Table 6.1. Once we have imported the data, we need to divide our data points into training and testing subsets. We randomly assign data points to training and testing groups, and we make the classification model based on the training data. In order to assess how good our model is in predicting the class of a data point, we employ the model to classify the data points assigned to the testing group.

Before assigning our data points to training and testing groups, we need to understand the structure of our data set, and make the necessary changes:

```
> str(data)
'data.frame':   30 obs. of  4 variables:
 $ Regimen      : chr  "A" "C" "A" "B" ...
 $ TAM          : chr  "M1" "M1" "M2" "M1" ...
 $ Increased.MMP: chr  "Yes" "No" "Yes" "Yes" ...
 $ Survival     : chr  "Intermediate" "Long" "Short" "Long" ...
```

As can be seen, R is reading our features as characters; however, in order to be able to use the variables to create the model, we need to turn these variables into factors:

```
> data$Regimen<- as.factor(data$Regimen)
> data$TAM <- as.factor(data$TAM)
> data$Increased.MMP <- as.factor(data$Increased.MMP)
> data$Survival <- as.factor(data$Survival)
```

Now, let us plot our data to get an idea of the distribution of the data points. We can also find if the assumption of Naïve Bayes', independence of independent variables, is met. In order to plot the data points, we use the "psych" package [6]:

```
> install.packages("psych")
> library(psych)
```

As can be seen in Fig. 6.1, independent variables are not strongly correlated, which allows us to use Naïve Bayes' for classification. It is important to remember that even if the assumption of independence of covariates does not hold true, we can still use Naïve Bayes' for the classification of our observations; however, the performance of our model will be compromised due to non-conformity to its assumptions.

Now, we can assign these data points to training and testing groups. In order to make the results reproducible, we set the seed to a specific number, so the process of randomly assigning data points to the training and testing groups does not affect the results we get each time we run the model:

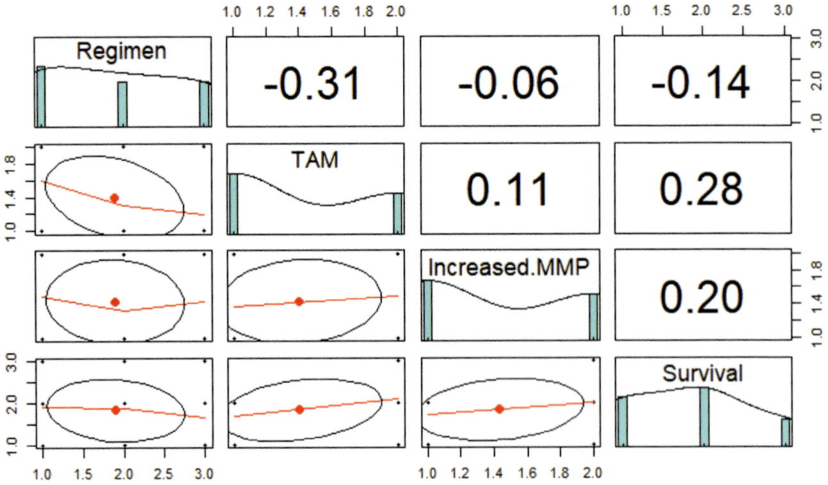

FIGURE 6.1 Distribution plot of data.

```
> set.seed(123)
> subsets <- sample(2, nrow(data), prob=c(0.7, 0.3), replace=T)
> train <- data[subsets==1,]
> test <- data[subsets==2,]
```

Now let us train our model using the training subset of our data. We need to first install and call the necessary package to create a Naïve Bayes' model:

```
> install.packages("naivebayes")
> library(naivebayes)
> NB_Model<- naive_bayes(data$Survival ~ data$Regimen + data$TAM + data$Incre
ased.MMP, data=train)
Warning messages:
1: naive_bayes(): Feature data$TAM - zero probabilities are present. Consider
Laplace smoothing.
2: naive_bayes(): Feature data$Increased.MMP - zero probabilities are present
. Consider Laplace smoothing.
```

As mentioned earlier, a small data set can pose certain challenges. One of these challenges is that certain combinations of features and class variables are not present in the training set, resulting in zero probability of that event in the training set. However, as indicated by R, this can be taken care of by Laplace smoothing.

Laplace smoothing, also known as Laplace correction, is a method of overcoming zero probabilities, or zero frequencies, reserved for categorical variables, as zero probability only occurs with categorical variables. In order to overcome the zero-frequency issue, in Laplace smoothing we add a certain value to the numerator of all probabilities used in Bayes' rule; this way, we can avoid zero occurrence. Even though any constant can be chosen for Laplace smoothing, the smaller the number is, the closer the probabilities are to real probabilities. This will be further explained while training Naïve Bayes' classifiers using the second data set in this chapter. In order to implement Laplace smoothing in R, we need to set the "laplace" argument in the "naïve_bayes" function to a number of our choice. Let us add 3 to the numerators:

```
> NB_Model<- naive_bayes(data$Survival ~ ., data=train, laplace = 3)
```

Now, let us summarize our classification model:

```
> NB_Model

============================================== Naive Bayes ===================
==========================

 Call:
naive_bayes.formula(formula = data$Survival ~ data$Regimen +
    data$TAM + data$Increased.MMP, data = train, laplace = 3)

------------------------------------------------------------------------------
--------------------------

Laplace smoothing: 3

------------------------------------------------------------------------------
--------------------------

 A priori probabilities:

Intermediate         Long        Short
   0.3666667    0.4333333    0.2000000

------------------------------------------------------------------------------
--------------------------

 Tables:

------------------------------------------------------------------------------
--------------------------
 ::: data$Regimen (Categorical)
------------------------------------------------------------------------------
--------------------------

data$Regimen Intermediate      Long     Short
           A    0.4000000 0.2727273 0.4666667
           B    0.2500000 0.4090909 0.2666667
           C    0.3500000 0.3181818 0.2666667
------------------------------------------------------------------------------
--------------------------
 ::: data$TAM (Bernoulli)
------------------------------------------------------------------------------
--------------------------

data$TAM Intermediate      Long     Short
      M1    0.5294118 0.7894737 0.2500000
      M2    0.4705882 0.2105263 0.7500000

------------------------------------------------------------------------------
--------------------------
 ::: data$Increased.MMP (Bernoulli)
------------------------------------------------------------------------------
--------------------------

data$Increased.MMP Intermediate      Long     Short
                No    0.4705882 0.7894737 0.2500000
               Yes    0.5294118 0.2105263 0.7500000

------------------------------------------------------------------------------
--------------------------
```

As can be seen, the probabilities are calculated for the class variables versus each of the independent variables. Expectedly, the class with the highest probability will be chosen as the class for the data set.

Even though Laplace correction helped us create the classification model, there are other issues with creating a predictive model based on a small data set, specifically if the correlations between the independent variables and the class variable are low. One such issue is that none of the independent variables can be a good predictor of the dependent variable as their association is loose. Let us assess the predictive accuracy of the model based on our data set:

```
> prediction <- predict(NB_Model, test)
Warning messages:
1: predict.naive_bayes(): only 0 feature(s) out of 3 defined in the naive_bay
es object "NB_Model" are used for prediction.

2: predict.naive_bayes(): more features in the newdata are provided as there
are probability tables in the object. Calculation is performed based on featu
res to be found in the tables.
3: predict.naive_bayes(): no feature in the newdata corresponds to probabilit
y tables in the object. Classification is done based on the prior probabiliti
es
```

The problem of loose association is encountered here, and as a result, the predictions are made only based on the prior probabilities of the class variable. In order to better understand the classification performance of the model, let us take a look at the confusion matrix:

```
> confusion_matrix <- table(prediction, test$Survival)
> confusion_matrix

prediction     Intermediate Long Short
  Intermediate            0    0     0
  Long                    3    6     1
  Short                   0    0     0
```

We now compare these with the frequency of each class in the test group:

```
> sum(test$Survival=="Long")
[1] 6
> sum(test$Survival=="Intermediate")
[1] 3
> sum(test$Survival=="Short")
[1] 1
```

As was mentioned when predicting classes, only the prior probabilities are used for the classification of the dependent variable.

We now move on to creating Naïve Bayes' classifier using our second data set, which will be used in future chapters as well. This data set, as presented in Table 6.2, represents the survival of neuroblastoma patients

TABLE 6.2 Neuroblastoma patients' characteristics and survival.

Age	Stage	Ki67 index (%)	p53	Survival
42	3	78	6	Intermediate
2	1	12	0	Long
34	2	46	2	Long
Age	Stage	Ki67 index	P53	Survival
6	2	63	11	Long
32	2	83	23	Short
15	4	80	28	Short
65	2	15	1	Long
23	4	78	13	Intermediate
63	3	51	0	Long
13	2	46	1	Intermediate
19	1	27	4	Long
54	2	58	11	Long
72	4	39	13	Intermediate
3	3	71	26	Short
14	3	62	21	Intermediate
56	2	18	1	Long
2	1	45	4	Long
43	4	58	23	Short
16	2	14	1	Long
17	3	71	12	Intermediate
52	2	64	5	Long
17	2	23	0	Long
26	2	89	0	Short
53	1	23	14	Long
1	1	10	0	Long
52	1	6	0	Long
71	3	41	2	Intermediate
4	4	78	21	Short
15	2	23	11	Long
67	1	15	4	Long
3	3	64	19	Short
46	3	48	3	Intermediate
17	2	23	0	Long
65	4	61	19	Long
37	1	11	0	Long
12	3	39	12	Short

based on features such as patients' age, their stage of the disease, and some other genetic factors. We need to check the structure of the data before dividing our data set into training and testing subsets:

```
> str(data)
'data.frame':     36 obs. of  5 variables:
 $ Age          : int  42 2 34 6 32 15 65 23 63 13 ...
 $ Stage        : int  3 1 2 2 2 4 2 4 3 2 ...
 $ Ki67.index....: int  78 12 46 63 83 80 15 78 51 46 ...
 $ p53          : int  6 0 2 11 23 28 1 13 0 1 ...
 $ Survival     : chr  "Intermediate" "Long" "Long" "Long" ...
```

As we know, cancer stage is a categorical data, so is the survival of the patients. Therefore, we need to change the class of these two variables:

```
> data$Stage <- as.factor((data$Stage))
> data$Survival <- as.factor(data$Survival)
```

Now, we can divide our data set into training and testing subsets:

```
> subsets <- sample(2, nrow(data), prob=c(0.7, 0.3), replace=T)
> train <- data[subsets==1,]
> test <- data[subsets==2,]
```

We use the same methods that were used to develop the first Naïve Bayes' classifier in this chapter; however, we delve deeper into the effect of parameters to train the model on its performance; therefore, we create multiple Naïve Bayes' classifiers using this data set.

For the first classifier, we do not use the Laplace smoothing method, and allow some of the probabilities to remain zero:

```
> NB1 <- naive_bayes(Survival~., data=train)
Warning message:
naive_bayes(): Feature Stage - zero probabilities are present. Consider
Laplace smoothing.
```

Now that we have trained our classifier, we move on to predicting patients' survival category in the testing subset of the data:

```
> prediction1 <- predict(NB1, test)
Warning message:
predict.naive_bayes(): more features in the newdata are provided as there are
probability tables in the object. Calculation is performed based on features
to be found in the tables.
```

The warning messages returned are inherent to the package used to train the data, and do not denote issues in our model. We should now make our confusion matrix to find the accuracy of the model in predicting the class of observations in the testing subset. We can use the confusionMatrix() function from the "caret" package for this purpose as it provides more information regarding our model's performance and the reliability on the numbers returned to represent the accuracy of the model:

```
> library(caret)
> ConfusionMatrix1 <- confusionMatrix(prediction1, test$Survival)
> ConfusionMatrix1
Confusion Matrix and Statistics

              Reference
Prediction     Intermediate Long Short
  Intermediate            1    1     0
  Long                    0    6     0
  Short                   2    1     2

Overall Statistics

               Accuracy : 0.6923
                 95% CI : (0.3857, 0.9091)
    No Information Rate : 0.6154
    P-Value [Acc > NIR] : 0.3966

                  Kappa : 0.5048

 Mcnemar's Test P-Value : 0.2615

Statistics by Class:

                     Class: Intermediate Class: Long Class: Short
Sensitivity                      0.33333      0.7500       1.0000
Specificity                      0.90000      1.0000       0.7273
Pos Pred Value                   0.50000      1.0000       0.4000
Neg Pred Value                   0.81818      0.7143       1.0000
Prevalence                       0.23077      0.6154       0.1538
Detection Rate                   0.07692      0.4615       0.1538
Detection Prevalence             0.15385      0.4615       0.3846
Balanced Accuracy                0.61667      0.8750       0.8636
```

The confusion matrix shows the types of misclassification, which can be helpful to observe if there is any inclination toward a specific category in predictions of our model, along with other important information. Accuracy of the model, here approximately 69%, is calculated by dividing the correct classification by the total number of the observations. No information rate shows us what percentage of observations are made up by the most common class of dependent variables. If these classes are disproportionate, there is a high chance that our model can be biased toward favoring one class over another in making predictions, if the data set is not large enough for the model to learn the patterns. An important aspect to be considered when evaluating the accuracy of a classifier is the *P*-value of the accuracy. In this case, *P*-value [Acc > NIR] for increased accuracy compared to no information rate is above the usual alpha threshold of significance, 0.05. This means that our model's accuracy is not significantly better than a map model, and the accuracy is not significantly higher than no information rate. In this model, no information rate is 61%, and the model's accuracy is 69%. The *P*-value of 0.39 shows that our model has only a 39% chance of outperforming a map model, which assigns classes to observations randomly. Another criterion to judge the performance of a classifier is the Kappa coefficient. Kappa coefficient shows how better our model is in making predictions compared to a map model, and this coefficient ranges between −1 and 1. Kappa of zero denotes the model has the same performance as a map model, Kappa less than zero shows that random assigning of classes is better than our model, and Kappa greater than zero shows our model outperforms a map model. McNemar's test *P*-value also shows that our model is not significantly better than the map model. To summarize our evaluation of the model's performance, we can say that even though the accuracy of the model is around 70%, which is considerable, the model's accuracy is not reliable based on the complementary information in the output.

There are several ways of attempting to improve the accuracy of our predictions: we can change the parameters of our model or we can choose to try different machine learning algorithms. However, the problem is we cannot increase our sample size, which can, otherwise, improve our model's performance. We will learn about other classification and regression models in future chapters. However, let us briefly overview the effects of a model's parameters on its performance, while focusing on Laplace smoothing.

We mentioned earlier that the smaller the constant assigned to the "laplace" argument in the naivebayes() function is, the better the performance of the model will be. This is due to the fact that the constant added to the numerators to compose probabilities will be closer to the real numerators, so the probabilities are closer to real proportions of observations in the data set. To better understand this effect, we train two Naïve Bayes' classifiers, NB2 and NB3, using the nuroblastoma patient's survival table.

```
> NB2 <- naive_bayes(Survival~., data=train, laplace=5)
> prediction2 <- predict(NB2, test)
Warning message:
predict.naive_bayes(): more features in the newdata are provided as there are
probability tables in the object. Calculation is performed based on features
to be found in the tables.
> ConfusionMatrix_NB2 <- confusionMatrix(prediction2, test$Survival)
> ConfusionMatrix_NB2
Confusion Matrix and Statistics

              Reference
Prediction     Intermediate Long Short
  Intermediate            0    3     0
  Long                    1    4     0
  Short                   2    1     2

Overall Statistics

               Accuracy : 0.4615
                 95% CI : (0.1922, 0.7487)
    No Information Rate : 0.6154
    P-Value [Acc > NIR] : 0.9211

                  Kappa : 0.1727

 Mcnemar's Test P-Value : 0.2615

Statistics by Class:

                     Class: Intermediate Class: Long Class: Short
Sensitivity                       0.0000      0.5000       1.0000
Specificity                       0.7000      0.8000       0.7273
Pos Pred Value                    0.0000      0.8000       0.4000
Neg Pred Value                    0.7000      0.5000       1.0000
Prevalence                        0.2308      0.6154       0.1538
Detection Rate                    0.0000      0.3077       0.1538
Detection Prevalence              0.2308      0.3846       0.3846
Balanced Accuracy                 0.3500      0.6500       0.8636
```

All the statistics, including accuracy, *P*-value of accuracy, and Kappa coefficient, show that this model is not better than NB1, for which Laplace smoothing was not performed. We move on with creating our third classifier:

```
> NB3 <- naive_bayes(Survival~., data=train, laplace=3)

> prediction3 <- predict(NB3, test)

Warning message:

predict.naive_bayes(): more features in the newdata are provided as there are
probability tables in the object. Calculation is performed based on features
to be found in the tables.

> ConfusionMatrix_NB3 <- confusionMatrix(prediction3, test$Survival)

> ConfusionMatrix_NB3

Confusion Matrix and Statistics


              Reference

Prediction     Intermediate Long Short

  Intermediate            0    2     0

  Long                    1    5     0

  Short                   2    1     2


Overall Statistics


               Accuracy : 0.5385

                 95% CI : (0.2513, 0.8078)

    No Information Rate : 0.6154

    P-Value [Acc > NIR] : 0.8051


                  Kappa : 0.2571


 Mcnemar's Test P-Value : 0.3430


Statistics by Class:


                    Class: Intermediate Class: Long Class: Short

Sensitivity                      0.0000      0.6250       1.0000

Specificity                      0.8000      0.8000       0.7273

Pos Pred Value                   0.0000      0.8333       0.4000

Neg Pred Value                   0.7273      0.5714       1.0000

Prevalence                       0.2308      0.6154       0.1538

Detection Rate                   0.0000      0.3846       0.1538

Detection Prevalence             0.1538      0.4615       0.3846

Balanced Accuracy                0.4000      0.7125       0.8636
```

Comparing the results from the three classifiers, we can conclude that even though some show improved performance when comparing accuracy percentage, none of these classifiers show a substantially reliable accuracy as the P-values for the three models are greater than alpha threshold of 0.05. There are a few reasons behind this observation. One of them is the small training and testing subsets. Another reason is the proportion of classes, or prior probability, in the training and testing subsets. Additionally, Bayes algorithm is not the best algorithm to train models based on small data sets. In future chapters, we will learn about other classifiers that can help us improve our predictions as each algorithm is best suitable for a specific type of data structure.

References

[1] J.L. Puga, M. Krzywinski, N. Altman, Points of significance: Bayes' theorem, Nature Methods 12 (4) (2015) 277–278. Available from: https://doi.org/10.1038/nmeth.3335.

[2] J. Wolfson, S. Bandyopadhyay, M. Elidrisi, G. Vazquez-Benitez, D.M. Vock, D. Musgrove, et al., A Naive Bayes machine learning approach to risk prediction using censored, time-to-event data, Statistics in Medicine 34 (21) (2015) 2941–2957. Available from: https://doi.org/10.1002/sim.6526.

[3] A. Benavoli, C. de Campos, Bayesian dependence tests for continuous, binary and mixed continuous-binary variables, Entropy 18 (9) (2016) 326. Available from: https://doi.org/10.3390/e18090326.

[4] F. Fischer, Using Bayes theorem to estimate positive and negative predictive values for continuously and ordinally scaled diagnostic tests, International Journal of Methods in Psychiatric Research 30 (2) (2021) e1868. Available from: https://doi.org/10.1002/mpr.1868.

[5] J.A. Bittl, Y. He, Bayesian analysis: a practical approach to interpret clinical trials and create clinical practice guidelines, Circulation: Cardiovascular Quality and Outcomes 10 (8) (2017). Available from: https://doi.org/10.1161/CIRCOUTCOMES.117.003563.

[6] R. Revelle, Psych: Procedures for Psychological, Psychometric, and Personality Research, 2021.

CHAPTER

7

Linear and logistic regressions in R

What is regression?

The term regression, in the concept being introduced here, was first used in the 19th century following the observation that the offspring of parents with extremely short or extremely tall statures tend to have statures closer to average and hence the term "regression to the mean" [1]. In statistics, methods by which we analyze the relationship between a dependent variable (the outcome) and one or more independent variables or covariates are called regression methods [2]. Regression analysis encompasses a large number of methods dedicated to analyzing such relationships. There are various regression models that can be used either for making numeric predictions such as the linear regression for continuous data [2] or Poisson regression for integer count data [3] or for classification purposes such as logistic regression [4]. In previous chapters, we overviewed data structures and how understanding the relationship between different features and the outcome can help us build models that can predict the outcome for unseen data.

In this chapter, we will learn about two types of regression for the prediction of continuous and categorical data: linear and logistic regressions, respectively.

Linear regression

Linear regression deals with the prediction of continuous numeric outcomes, and it is most commonly used to investigate the relationship between two quantitative variables [2]. Given their properties in making numeric prediction, linear regression models have numerous

Immunoinformatics of Cancers
DOI: https://doi.org/10.1016/B978-0-12-822400-7.00004-X

applications in medicine and bioinformatics, similar to other scientific fields. A few of these applications include the prediction of patients' survival based on gene expression levels or other characteristics and prediction of gene expression patterns in cell reprogramming [5], among several others [6].

Linear regression algorithms have some key assumptions. These assumptions must be met in order to use the linear regression algorithms, or at least for linear regression algorithm to yield acceptable results [2]. The first assumption is that our data follow a linear trend. This can be inferred from the scatter plot of the data points. The second assumption is that a linear combination of the independent variables follows a normal distribution. This can be verified using the Q–Q plots of the variables. The third assumption is that there should not be a high level of correlation, or multicollinearity, among the independent variables. Furthermore, there should not be a high level of residual dependency in the data. The final assumption is homoscedasticity of the data, meaning that the residuals on the sides of the fit line are approximately equal. However, there can be some robustness to deviation from any of these assumptions.

In Chapter 5, we mentioned that one of the simplest forms of predictive models is the one that tries to delineate the relationship between the outcome and the independent variable with a straight line. The line follows a polynomial expression, which in the simplest form of modeling factors in only one independent variable to predict the outcome (dependent variable) [2]:

$$y = ax + c \tag{7.1}$$

In fact, linear regression investigates whether there is a linear relationship between two or more variables. Therefore, building a linear model is about finding the slope (a) and the intercept (c) in a way that the created line returns a y (outcome) for any given x (input) that is closest to the actual corresponding y of that given input [2]. As this line is extremely unlikely to explain all the data points in our observations, we need to add an error term or a residual (ε_i), which equals the difference between the actual outcome (y) in that point and the predicted outcome (y_i) for that point [2].

$$y = ax + c + \varepsilon_i \tag{7.2}$$

Here, a can be any real number and indicates the amount of change in y (outcome) for every unit of change in the independent variable. An a of greater than zero ($a > 0$) indicates a direct relationship between the target variable (outcome) and the predictive variables (independent features) and negative a values indicate a negative correlation between the dependent and the independent variables. An a of zero is interpreted as a lack of linear correlation between the dependent and independent variables [2].

Simple linear regression factors in only one variable to build the predictive model; however, in a more complicated model, more features are factored in to build the model [2]. Bear in mind that as long as the model follows a first-degree polynomial expression, the predictive model remains a straight line (multiple linear regression).

The fact that y is dependent of x makes linear regression a form of conditional expectation. Before we discuss conditional expectation, let us go over the concept of expected value.

Expected value

One of the important concepts of probability that can be seen in various machine learning algorithms is the concept of expected value. Any random feature is associated with a probability distribution that determines the rate of occurrence for that feature. There are different distributions of probability, the most common being the normal distribution, which we might know as the bell-shaped or the standard distribution. Expected value of a random variable is a measure of its average or the value typically observed for that variable and is shown by $E[x]$ [7]. The expected value for each variable is the sum of the product of each outcome and its probability:

$$E[x] = \sum_{x} x \times p(x) \tag{7.3}$$

where x is the outcome and $p(x)$ is the probability of that outcome. As an instance, consider the frequency of MYCN mutation among neuroblastoma patients is 20%. Therefore, the probability (p) of MYCN mutation is 0.2; hence, the probability of not having this mutation among neuroblastoma patients is ($1-p$), which equals 0.8. This type of random variable with only two outcomes is called a Bernoulli random variable. In a Bernoulli random variable, the occurrence of an event ("success") is labeled 1 and failure is labeled 0. Based on Eq. (7.1), the expected value for MYCN mutation among neuroblastoma patients is given by

$$E[x] = (1 \times p) + (0 \times (1-p))$$

$$E[MYCN\ mutation] = (1 \times 0.2) + (0 \times 0.8) = 0.2$$

As a general rule, the expected value for a Bernoulli random variable is equal to the "success" probability.

Linear regression can be considered as a conditional expectation, meaning estimating the probability of occurrence of event Y given that the event X has occurred. This can be expressed by the following equation:

$$E[Y|X] = ax + c \tag{7.4}$$

Similar to Eq. (7.1), Eq. (7.4) denotes that 1 unit of increase in X leads to a units of increase in Y. As mentioned earlier, the aim of linear regression is to find the a and c parameters in a way that the line representing the model passes as close as possible to all data points. The measure of this closeness is known as ordinary least-squares, which is the sum of the squared residuals. The residuals are the difference between the actual outcome for each instance in the data and the predicted value for that incidence by the model (Fig. 7.1).

$$\varepsilon_i = \hat{y} - y_i \tag{7.5}$$

where ε_i is the residual, $\hat{y}$ is the predicted outcome, and y is the actual outcome. In order to avoid negative values, the sum of squared residuals or the sum of squared estimate of errors for each data point is used as a measure for efficiency of the predictive model. Residual sum of squares is calculated as

$$\text{RSS} = \sum_{i=1}^{n} \varepsilon_i^2 = \sum_{i=1}^{n} (\hat{y} - y_i)^2 \tag{7.6}$$

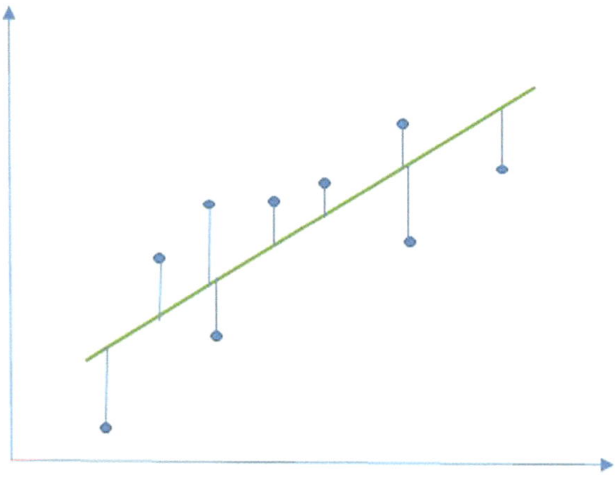

FIGURE 7.1 Graph of the linear fit and the residuals.

The aim of a good predictive model is to choose the parameters, that is, the intercept and slope, in a way that a residual sum of squares (RSS) as small as possible is returned. The intercept (c in Eqs. 7.1 and 7.3) can be obtained by using the following equation:

$$c = \overline{Y} - \alpha\overline{X} \tag{7.7}$$

where $\overline{Y}$ is the sample mean of the outcomes and $\overline{X}$ is the sample mean of features. However, as can be noted, in order to find this intercept, we need to know the slope, which is calculated as

$$\alpha = \frac{\sum_{i=1}^{n}(x_i - \overline{X})(y_i - \overline{Y})}{\sum_{i=1}^{n}(x_i - \overline{X})^2} \tag{7.8}$$

Multiple regression

Many of the data sets we deal with in life sciences provide information regarding multiple factors and their relation to our target variable. Linear regression can be used to determine the relation between the multiple factors included in a data set and investigate their relationship to the outcome.

$$y_i = \alpha + \beta_1 x_i^1 + \beta_2 x_i^2 + \cdots + \beta_k x_i^k + \varepsilon_i \tag{7.9}$$

However, as can be expected, the calculations to determine the coefficients and other parameters of the model are more complicated and time-consuming than simple linear regression. Luckily, we do not need to worry about these calculations as R handles them for us; therefore, if you are not interested in the mathematics behind the process of finding the model parameters, you can simply ignore the formulas. Now that we have a fair insight into how a linear regression model is built, let us see how we can use R to build a linear regression model for us.

Hands-on linear regression with R

As mentioned before, one of the most important factors that lead us to choosing one machine learning algorithm over another is the structure of the data at hand. For our purposes of learning how to build linear regression with R, consider the example data set below on survival of neuroblastoma patients based on patients' characteristics such as age, as well as the molecular features of the tumor, such as Ki-67 and p53 expression. Table 7.1 presents the data set on survival of the neuroblastoma patients and their characteristics.

TABLE 7.1 Example data on survival of neuroblastoma patients.

Age	Stage	Ki67 index (%)	p53	Survival
42	3	78	6	13
2	1	12	0	102
34	2	46	2	43
6	2	63	11	12
32	2	83	23	5
15	4	80	28	1
65	2	15	1	45
23	4	78	13	7
63	3	51	0	41
13	2	46	1	23
19	1	27	4	45
54	2	58	11	32
72	4	39	13	14
3	3	71	26	6
14	3	62	21	13
56	2	18	1	56
2	1	45	4	33
43	4	58	23	9
16	2	14	1	45
17	3	71	12	18
52	2	64	5	41
17	2	23	0	76
26	2	89	0	4
53	1	23	14	37
1	1	10	0	94
52	1	6	0	65
71	3	41	2	19

(Continued)

TABLE 7.1 (Continued)

Age	Stage	Ki67 index (%)	p53	Survival
4	4	78	21	5
15	2	23	11	43
67	1	15	4	27
3	3	64	19	9
46	3	48	3	14
17	2	23	0	56
65	4	61	19	7
37	1	11	0	93
12	3	39	12	9

One of the first steps in creating any model explaining the relationship between different variables of a data set is visualizing these relationships. There are various ways to demonstrate this relationship, including, but not limited to, correlation matrix, density plots, and scatter plots. But how can we understand the relations between variables from the scatter plots?

To answer this question, let us first explain what a scatter plot is: A scatter plot is a plot that shows values of two different variables in the form of dots in a two-dimensional coordinate. If the values for one variable increase with increase in the values for the other variables, these two variables have a direct relationship, and if the values of one variable increase with decrease in the values for the other variables, these variables have an inverse relationship or a negative correlation. Examples of direct and inverse linear relationships between two variables are demonstrated in Fig. 7.2. Even though the scatter plots in Fig. 7.2 are rather simplistic and we often do not encounter such straightforward linear relationships between variables, we must bear in mind that as long as a straight line can be fitted to the data points, we can explain the relationship between the variables with simple linear regression. However, as linear models ignore all other forms of relationship between the data points, they may not be the best model to explain the relationship between variables. By inspecting the scatter plot of the data points, it is possible to predict whether

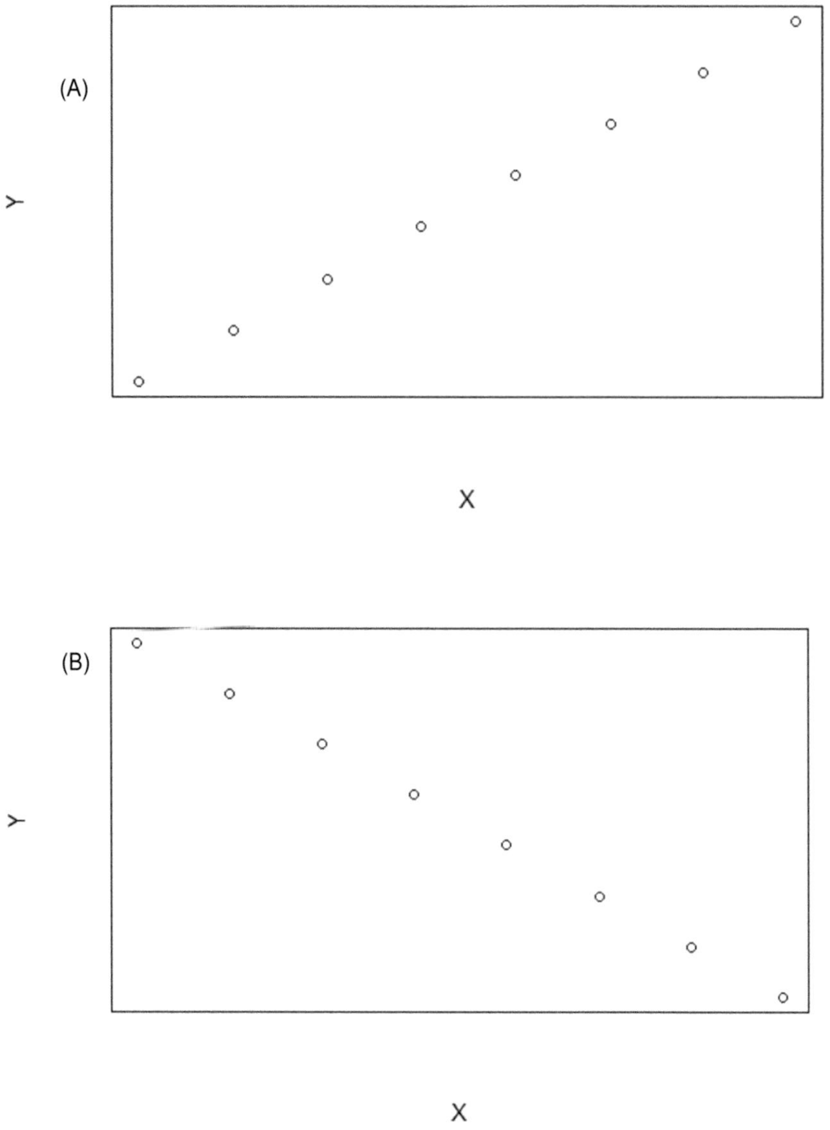

FIGURE 7.2 (A) Variables X and Y have a direct linear relationship. As the values of X increase, values of Y increase as well. (B) Variables X and Y have an inverse linear relationship. As the values of X increase, values of Y decrease.

a linear regression is a good model to explain the relationships in our data set. For this purpose, let us visualize the relationship between the independent variables and the target variable (survival) in Table 7.1.

NOTE...

We can attempt to find the best models explaining the relationship between the data points. This can be achieved by increasing the parameters involved in our predictive model and defining several conditions. However, this can be at the expense of time, memory, and complexity of the model. Another downfall of making a highly complex model is overfitting, as discussed in previous chapters. This also will make the model less accurate when facing new data [8]. As we mentioned, one of the main goals of machine learning is to make predictions on new data. If our model is extremely complex, it compromises its applicability for other data sets.

Another important aspect of developing predictive algorithms is that the accuracy of the model can be increased only to a certain level by adjusting the parameters involved in the model, such as feature selection discussed in previous chapters. This leaves the data set and the nature of the relationship among the variables as the main factor influencing how accurate a model can be. And how well a model can predict the outcomes of a new data set depends to a great extent on whether the new data set has the same pattern of relationship between its components as the data set the model was trained upon.

Various functions can be used to view the scatter plot of different variables. Obviously, the scatter plots obtained using either of the available functions will be generally the same; however, some of these functions return the correlation coefficient and the density plots as well. Some of these functions are built-in, while others, which usually provide more complicated plots, belong to specific R packages. We will review some of these functions to get the scatter plots of the data presented in Table 7.1.

Two of the built-in functions returning the simplest forms of scatter plots are the pairs() function and the plot() function. Using either of these functions will result in the plot presented in Fig. 7.2.

```
# getting the plot of the data
> plot(table1)
Or
> pairs(table1)
```

Even though it is possible to fit a line to the data points in any data set, regardless of their distribution, it is obvious that some of the relationships between different variables are not best explained by a linear regression. In the scatter plots presented in Fig. 7.3, the relationship between each two sets of variables is demonstrated by the scatter plots at their respective intersections. For instance, the relationship between

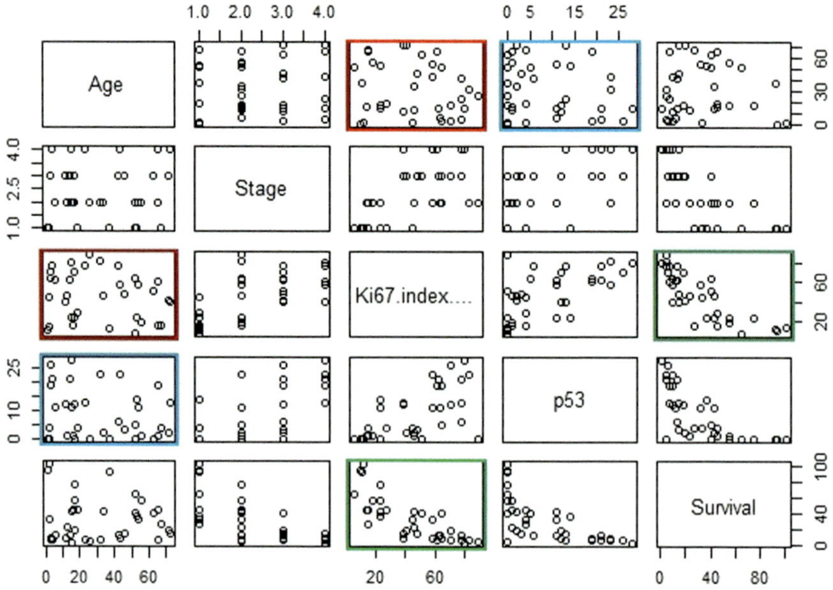

FIGURE 7.3 Scatter plot of the relation between different variables presented in Table 7.1. The scatter plots in red boxes demonstrate the relationship between Ki67 index and age, the scatter plots in blue boxes show the relationship between p53 and age, and the scatter plots in green boxes show the relationship between Ki67 index and survival.

Ki67 index and the survival is an inverse relationship. This relationship can be explained by a linear regression, even though this may not be the best way to explain their relationship. In the same figure, the relationship between age and either Ki67 index or p53 is more scattered in comparison to the relationship between survival and Ki67 index. As it is not practical to fit a line to the data points of categorical variables, it is difficult to understand the relationship between two categorical variables or the relationship between categorical and numerical variables. However, R can determine the effect of categorical variables by determining their correlation coefficients.

A more complicated plot provided by the "psych" package [9] returns not only the scatter plots, but also the correlation coefficients as well as the density plot. Let us use this package to demonstrate these plots for the data presented in Table 7.1:

```
# getting a more detailed plot of the data
> install.packages("psych")
> library(psych)
> pairs.panels(table1)
```

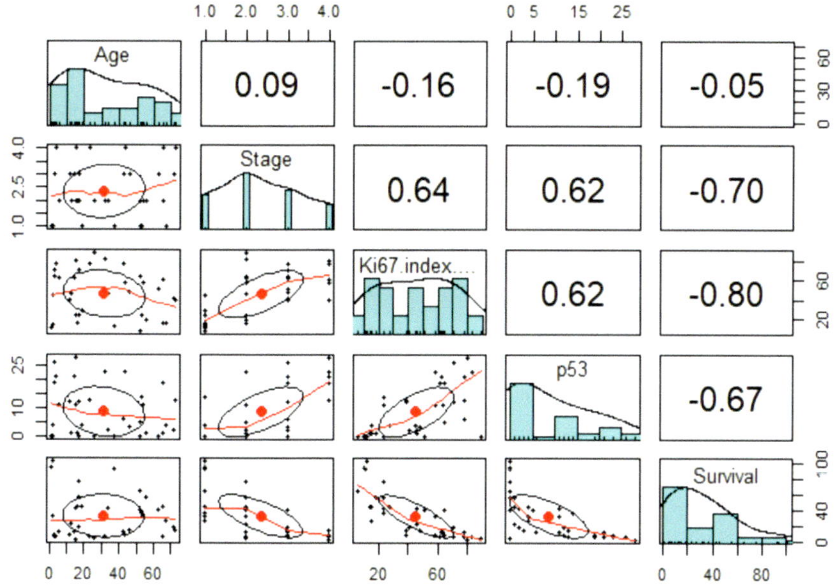

FIGURE 7.4 Scatter plots and the correlation coefficients demonstrating the relationship between different variables. Density plots show the distribution of each variable, which can be used to determine whether a variable has a normal distribution.

The code will give us the matrix of plots and correlation coefficients shown in Fig. 7.4. From this matrix, we can have a rough estimate of the hyperparameters of our model. For instance, the higher the correlation coefficient of an independent variable is, the higher the coefficient parameter of that variable will be in our final model.

Now let us learn how to build the model using the built-in R function, `lm()`, using the data presented in Table 7.1. In order to build a linear regression model, which in our case will be a multiple linear regression due to the number of independent variables, we must first determine whether the size of our data set is appropriate for the number of variables we aim to include in our model. As mentioned before, a rule of thumb to determine the sample size required to build a model is roughly 10-fold the number of independent variables included in building the model. There are four independent variables (Age, Stage, Ki67 index, and p53 expression) associated with survival of neuroblastoma patients (the target or the dependent variable). Therefore, we require about 40 samples; however, we have 36 samples. We can either ignore this minor difference between the required and available samples or perform feature selection to include the most effective features. We will build two models using either of the methods and compare their performance. We will start by including all independent variables to create our first predictive model, then we will perform feature selection to create our second model.

Before we begin with creating the model, let us have a look at some general information about our data through the built-in R function, summary ():

```
> summary(table1)
      Age             Stage          Ki67.index....        p53              Survival
 Min.   : 1.00   Min.   :1.000   Min.   : 6.00   Min.   : 0.000   Min.   :  1.00
 1st Qu.:13.75   1st Qu.:2.000   1st Qu.:23.00   1st Qu.: 1.000   1st Qu.:  9.00
 Median :24.50   Median :2.000   Median :46.00   Median : 4.500   Median : 25.00
 Mean   :31.36   Mean   :2.361   Mean   :45.36   Mean   : 8.639   Mean   : 32.28
 3rd Qu.:52.25   3rd Qu.:3.000   3rd Qu.:64.00   3rd Qu.:13.250   3rd Qu.: 45.00
 Max.   :72.00   Max.   :4.000   Max.   :89.00   Max.   :28.000   Max.   :102.00
```

By now, we have an overall idea of the distribution of our data and the relationship between different components of the data set from the functions `summary()` and `plot()`. We must now "train" our model. For this purpose, we must divide our data set into training and testing subsets. In order for our results to be reproducible, we eliminate the effect of randomization using the R built-in function `set.seed()`. This will result in a repeatable division of data into testing and training subsets. We can choose any number for the `set.seed()` function; here, we choose 12.

```
> set.seed(123)
```

One of the easy ways of splitting a data set into testing and training subsets is using the `sample.split()` function from the "caTools" package [10]. We discussed the appropriate ratios for testing and training subsets in previous chapters. We choose the ratio of 7:3 for our training and testing models.

```
> install.packages("caTools")
> library(caTools)
> split_data=sample.split(table1, SplitRatio = 0.7)
```

Our data are now ready to be split into training and testing samples. For this purpose, we assign data points for which split is "TRUE" to training data:

```
> train=subset(table1, split_data="TRUE")
```

And then we define the test subset by choosing data points for which split is "FALSE":

```
> test=subset(table1, split_data="FALSE")
```

If we print test and train subsets, they look exactly like our original data set as we do not know which data point is assigned FALSE split or TRUE split:

```
> train
   Age Stage Ki67.index....p53 Survival
1   42     3              78   6       13
2    2     1              12   0      102
3   34     2              46   2       43
4    6     2              63  11       12
5   32     2              83  23        5
6   15     4              80  28        1
7   65     2              15   1       45
8   23     4              78  13        7
9   63     3              51   0       41
10  13     2              46   1       23
11  19     1              27   4       45
12  54     2              58  11       32
13  72     4              39  13       14
14   3     3              71  26        6
15  14     3              62  21       13
16  56     2              18   1       56
17   2     1              45   4       33
18  43     4              58  23        9
19  16     2              14   1       45
20  17     3              71  12       18
21  52     2              64   5       41
22  17     2              23   0       76
23  26     2              89   0        4
24  53     1              23  14       37
25   1     1              10   0       94
26  52     1               6   0       65
27  71     3              41   2       19
28   4     4              78  21        5
29  15     2              23  11       43
30  67     1              15   4       27
```

```
31   3      3                64  19          9
32  46      3                48   3         14
33  17      2                23   0         56
34  65      4                61  19          7
35  37      1                11   0         93
36  12      3                39  12          9
> test
   Age Stage Ki67.index.... p53 Survival
1   42     3             78   6       13
2    2     1             12   0      102
3   34     2             46   2       43
4    6     2             63  11       12
5   32     2             83  23        5
6   15     4             80  28        1
7   65     2             15   1       45
8   23     4             78  13        7
9   63     3             51   0       41
10  13     2             46   1       23
11  19     1             27   4       45
12  54     2             58  11       32
13  72     4             39  13       14
14   3     3             71  26        6
15  14     3             62  21       13
16  56     2             18   1       56
17   2     1             45   4       33
18  43     4             58  23        9
19  16     2             14   1       45
20  17     3             71  12       18
21  52     2             64   5       41
22  17     2             23   0       76
23  26     2             89   0        4
24  53     1             23  14       37
25   1     1             10   0       94
26  52     1              6   0       65
27  71     3             41   2       19
```

29	15	2	23	11	43
30	67	1	15	4	27
31	3	3	64	19	9
32	46	3	48	3	14
33	17	2	23	0	56
34	65	4	61	19	7
35	37	1	11	0	93
36	12	3	39	12	9

NOTE...

Another easy method to select sample size which requires no specific package is to define our train and test subsets and then select the corresponding rows from our data set. Here is how to define the train and test subsets for the data presented in Table 7.1:

```
> set.seed(12)
> N=nrow(table1)
```

As we wish to divide our data set by a proportion of 7:3, we allocate 25 data points to our training data and 15 data point to our testing data:

```
> train=sample(1:N, 25, FALSE)
> traindata=table1[train,]
> testdata=table1[-train,]
```

Now let us see if we got everything right:

```
> nrow(testdata)
[1] 11
> nrow(traindata)
[1] 25
```

All seems good, we have 25 training data points and 11 testing data points.

To have a better understanding of how the data set is being split into training and testing samples and what are the data points in each of these subsets, we use the R built-in function sample() to divide our data set into training and testing subsets.

```
> set.seed(123)
> subsets <- sample(2, nrow(data), prob=c(0.7, 0.3), replace=T)
> train <- data[subsets==1,]
> test <- data[subsets==2,]
```

Now we can create our model based on the training subset. Suppose we call our model "Model":

```
> Model <- lm(Survival~., data=train)
```

What is to the left of the "~" sign is our target variable, and if we do not determine the independent variables to the right side of the "~" sign and simply place a "." just like what we did in creating our model, the model will include all the independent variables in making the predictions. Now our model is built based on the training subset. We can see characteristics of our model through using the `summary()` function.

```
> summary(Model)

Call:
lm(formula = Survival ~ ., data = train)

Residuals:
    Min      1Q  Median      3Q     Max 
-25.469  -8.930  -0.089   7.402  29.742 

Coefficients:
                Estimate Std. Error t value Pr(>|t|)    
(Intercept)      81.8865    10.5535   7.759 3.78e-07 ***
Age              -0.2120     0.1622  -1.307  0.20767    
Stage            -3.8947     5.8992  -0.660  0.51749    
Ki67.index....   -0.6263     0.1851  -3.384  0.00331 ** 
p53              -0.7304     0.5832  -1.252  0.22643    
---
Signif. codes:  0 '***' 0.001 '**' 0.01 '*' 0.05 '.' 0.1 ' ' 1

Residual standard error: 16.12 on 18 degrees of freedom
Multiple R-squared:  0.7123,	Adjusted R-squared:  0.6484 
F-statistic: 11.14 on 4 and 18 DF,  p-value: 9.997e-05
```

The asterisks at the end of each variable line shows its significance in our predictive model, which is based on the last column of the table in the summary of the model, Pr. The line "`Signif. Codes`" helps us understand how to interpret these asterisks. In our model based on the data presented in Table 7.1, the most important independent variable is Ki67 index, and other variables do not contribute as much in making the predictive model.

Some statistics of our model that are indicative of its performance, such as R-squared and residual standard error, are mentioned in our model's summary. However, before we decide how well our model performs, we must see how closely it predicts the values of our testing subset. We also need to make sure that our model meets the criteria of a linear regression model. For this purpose, we check if our residuals follow a normal distribution. The density plot of residuals along with the Q–Q plot will give us a general idea of the normality of distributions for our model's residuals:

```
> plot(density(Model$residuals))
```

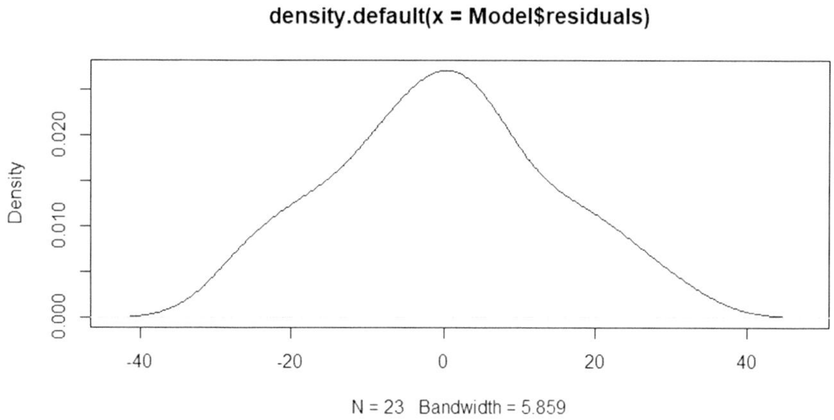

FIGURE 7.5 Density plot of residuals shows a normal distribution.

Fig. 7.5 shows the density plot of our model's residual distribution. This normality of distribution of errors is confirmed by the Q–Q plot shown in Fig. 7.6. To obtain the Q–Q plot of our model, along some additional plots, we use the R base function plot(), and y hitting "Return" in Console, we get the "Residuals vs. fitted" values, "Normal Q–Q," "Scale-Location," and Cook's distance in "Residuals vs. Leverage" plots.

```
> plot(Model)
Hit <Return> to see next plot:
```

As can be derived, the distribution of residuals is normal; however, we can be sure of the normality of distribution of residuals using a Shapiro–Wilk test through using the built-in function of R `shapiro.test()`. As the null hypothesis is that the distribution of residuals is normal, as long as we cannot rule out this hypothesis, it means that our residuals have a normal distribution.

```
> shapiro.test(Model$residuals)

        Shapiro-Wilk normality test

data:  Model$residuals
W = 0.98133, p-value = 0.7891
```

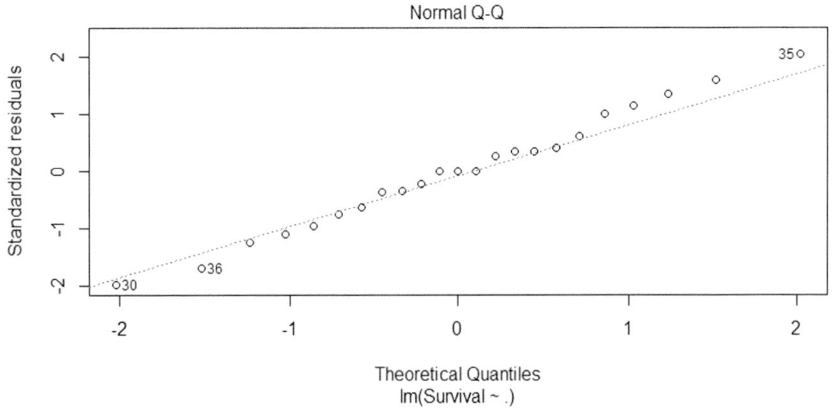

FIGURE 7.6 Q–Q plot of residuals showing a normal distribution of residuals. In this plot, residuals are plotted in an ascending order and are plotted against the expected quantiles from a normal distribution function.

Since the *P*-value for Shapiro test is above the normal alpha threshold (usually 0.05), we cannot rule out the null hypothesis and our residuals have a normal distribution. Now we can use our model to make predictions, first, on our test model, and if the model shows to be accurate, then on other relevant data. We call the values for our testing subset "prediction":

```
> predictions <- predict(Model, test)
> predictions
          2          4          5          8         11         16
20         21
70.0527222 25.3362448 -1.4664940  3.0879152 54.1328838 50.2211572
13.3689101 19.3398087
         24         26         31         32         34

42.1249701 63.2093873 15.6078857 28.1981629  0.4469031
```

Our goal now is to find out how deviated are these values from the actual values of our testing subset. In order to only assess the magnitude of this deviation and not let the direction of this deviation cloud our judgment on how good our model is, we attempt to remove the signs from the difference between the actual and predicted values by calculating the square root of the average of squared errors. This statistic is called root mean squared error (RMSE).

$$\text{RMSE} = \sqrt{\sum_{i=1}^{n} \frac{(\hat{y}_i - y_i)^2}{n}} \quad (7.10)$$

where $\hat{y}_i$ is the predicted value and y_i is the actual value. As is expected, the smaller the RMSE is, the more accurate our model is in predicting values. Let us calculate RMSE for predicting survival of the patients:

```
> rmse=sqrt(mean(predictions-test$Survival)^2)
> rmse
[1] 2.641503
```

As can be seen, the RMSE for our model is small compared to the magnitude of the target variable. But before making conclusions about the accuracy of our model, remember that we had mentioned that there are other statistics that in combination with RMSE determine the efficacy of our model. These statistics are residual standard error, F-statistics, and R-squared. Let us overview these statistics briefly.

Residual standard error

We introduced RMSE as a representative of the model's accuracy. To calculate RMSE, we divide the square of differences between the predicted values and actual values by the number of data points in our data set. Similarly, we can calculate residual standard error by dividing square of differences between predicated values and actual values by the degree of freedom:

$$\textit{residual standard error} = \sqrt{\sum_{i=1}^{n} \frac{(\hat{y}_i - y_i)^2}{df}} \quad (7.11)$$

where df is the degree of freedom. An advantage residual standard error has over RMSE is that it gives us an unbiased estimation of the deviation of the error term ε_i, as the degree of freedom varies with the number of the parameters we include in making our model. Similar to RMSE, a smaller residual standard error indicates better model accuracy in making predictions.

R-squared

One of the important parameters in determining the model's performance is R-squared (R^2) [11]. In the summary of the model we created based on data presented in Table 7.1, we can see that there are both "multiple R-squared" and "adjusted R-squared." The reason for providing both these values is that once we include multiple variables in creating our model, the performance of our model improves automatically compared to that of the mean model, which uses the mean for every predicted value once none of our predictor variables is informative.

An R-squared ranges between 0 and 1, and this number explains what percent of the changes in the dependent variables can be explained by the independent variables [11]. An R-squared of 0 means that our model has no advantage over the mean model and an R-squared of 1 means that our model perfectly predicts values. Predictions of our model improve as the number of independent variables included in the model increase. However, there are times when the ability of the model does not actually increase and the increase in R-squared is only due to the increase in the number of independent variables included in the model. This is why we need to adjust R-squared based on the number of independent variables of our model. However, this adjustment will not necessarily lead to decrease in R-squared. It only decreases R-squared if the number of the added independent variables does not make up for the decrease in degree of freedom. And if an addition of independent variables actually improves our model's predictions, this will lead to an increased adjusted R-squared. Therefore, in order to have a better understanding of our model's performance, we must always consider the adjusted R-squared when more than one independent variable is included in our model.

F-statistics

The F-test allows us to find out that whether an addition of more independent variables will lead to an improvement in the performance of our model in comparison to a model built based on no independent variable (also called intercept-only model). It also allows us to know if

R-squared is dependable or it is a random result of our data set. A significant F-test means that our model has better performance than an intercept-only model and that at least one of the independent variables affects the independent variable. However, remember that F-statistics is significant only if our *P*-values are below the alpha level (which is usually 0.05).

Considering the various factors determining a linear regression model's accuracy, the model created is of acceptable performance, but let us see if we can improve the performance of our model by choosing some of the features and eliminating the redundant or less important ones. As mentioned earlier, there are various methods for feature selection, and several R packages have been developed for each of these methods. We introduced one of the famous feature selection methods, principle component analysis (PCA), in Chapter 5. With the purpose of introducing as many feature selection methods as possible throughout this book, here we will introduce another method of feature selection. We use a package called "relaimpo" [12] to find the relative importance of each independent variable in our predictive model. This way we can use the independent variables with the highest relative importance and avoid unnecessary complexity of the model. To understand the relative importance of each of the independent variables, we can use the calc.relimp() function of the "relaimpo" package and sort them based on their relative importance:

```
> relative=calc.relimp(Model, type="lmg", rela=T)
> sort(relative$lmg, decreasing=T)
Ki67.index....       Stage         p53         Age
    0.47229893  0.26888204  0.22993844  0.02888058
```

As can be seen, Ki67 index is the most important predictive factor and the rest of the independent variables are similar in terms of importance in determining the outcome. This is where we need to rely on our own judgement and the information we have on the subject. In addition to the variables reported as important by various feature selection methods, we need to factor in background knowledge regarding the data and the nature of the relationship of the variables. Based on our general knowledge, we know that the stage of each cancer is one of the most important factors when it comes to predicting the outcome. This is backed up by the order of importance of independent variables, even though this importance is not significant compared to the importance of p53 and Age. We must now decide how many independent variables we want to include in our model. Let us include the maximum number of independent variables our sample size allows, which is three. We will exclude the least important feature, Age, and train our second model using the same training and testing data:

```
> Model2=lm(Survival~ Ki67.index.... + Stage + Stage, data=train)
> summary(Model2)

Call:
lm(formula = Survival ~ Ki67.index.... + Stage + Stage, data = train)

Residuals:
    Min      1Q  Median      3Q     Max
-37.104  -9.664  -2.896   7.295  26.814

Coefficients:
               Estimate Std. Error t value Pr(>|t|)
(Intercept)     82.9682     9.2398   8.979 1.87e-08 ***
Ki67.index....  -0.6164     0.1781  -3.461  0.00247 **
Stage           -9.6175     4.4220  -2.175  0.04181 *
---
Signif. codes:  0 '***' 0.001 '**' 0.01 '*' 0.05 '.' 0.1 ' ' 1

Residual standard error: 16.25 on 20 degrees of freedom
Multiple R-squared:  0.6752,    Adjusted R-squared:  0.6428
F-statistic: 20.79 on 2 and 20 DF,  p-value: 1.305e-05
> predict=predict(Model2, test)
> rmse=sqrt(mean(predict-test$Survival)^2)
> rmse
[1] 0.0552184
```

While multiple R-squared decreased, the adjusted R-squared remained the same, so our second model performs equally in covering the variability of the data as our first model. However, comparing the RMSE of the two models, we can conclude that the second model outperforms the first model. There are several reasons behind this improvement in predictions, one of which can be the increased ratio of training data points to the number of features. However, this might not always be the case as there are instances where decreasing the number of variables, especially if leads to exclusion of important features from training the model, can lead to decreased performance of the model. In such instances, the extent of the decrease in predictive abilities of the model must be weighed against the improvement in other parameters such as simplicity of the model as well as decreased time and memory required to make predictions [2,8].

Logistic regression

Logistic regression can be considered as an extension of linear regression, and, similar to linear regression, it belongs to the family of generalized linear models [4]. Originally, logistic regressions were developed to classify binary outcomes based on multiple categorical or continuous independent variables. Logistic regression makes these predictions based on probabilities obtained through maximum-likelihood estimations. As is expected, probability, denoted by $p(y)$, ranges between 0 and 1, with 0 assigned to the event not occurring and 1 assigned to the event occurring. Based on the probability estimated for each sample, which will be between 0 and 1, and the cutoff that we define for our model, logistic linear regression classifies samples into different groups. The probability cutoff for classifications depends on our purposes. For an instance, imagine we want to develop a logistic regression model to determine whether an individual has cancer or not. For this purpose, we define a lower cutoff of probability, say 0.4, for our model. This way our model is less likely to miss cancer cases by categorizing each patient with a probability of belonging to the cancer group, *p(cancer)*, that is, categorizing any probability greater than 0.4 as having cancer. However, it will be at the cost of performing unnecessary paraclinical studies to rule out cancer. Therefore, background knowledge is important in determining the cutoff value for our classification model.

Multinomial logistic regression is an extension of the classic binomial logistic regression, which allows making predictions regarding the classification of data points into more than two categories [4]. One the features that makes logistic regression one of the most favorite algorithms for classification purposes is that, unlike linear regression and many other classification algorithms based on ordinary least-squares, logistic regression does not have many assumptions about the data it deals with. Therefore, data that do not conform to assumptions of linearity, normality, and homoscedasticity can still be ideal to be classified using logistic regression.

We will briefly overview the mathematics behind the logistic regression algorithms. We will then move forward to hands-on examples of both types of regression using R.

Binomial logistic regression

When our target variable is binary, meaning that it can only have one of the two values, which are usually set to 1 when an event occurs or 0 when the event does not occur, our variable is called a binomial variable. For instance, consider we have some features of antigen-presenting cells and cytotoxic T cells such as their surface markers and we aim to classify our population of cells based on these features. We can arbitrarily assign two values to these cell types, so we assign cytotoxic T cells 1 and antigen-presenting cells 0. In general, we assign 0 to an event not occurring and 1 to when the event occurs. For example, imagine we aim to assign binary values to the occurrence of an event, such as response to treatment. In this case, we must set the occurrence of the event to 1, as in our calculations when we want to say that a patient has 100% (1 out of 1) chance of responding to treatment, the value we set to this event must reflect in our calculations. Similarly, when the patient has no chance of responding to treatment, the assigned value must reflect this chance, which is 0.

In order to make predictions about the occurrence of an event, we tend to find the probability of its occurrence based on previous patterns or other information we might have at hand. This way we can estimate the odds of an event occurring. For example, in the example of response to treatment, if out of the 1473 patients treated with a drug 1285 patients responded, then the odds of a patient responding to this drug is

$$Odds\ of\ response = \frac{Number\ of\ patients\ who\ responded\ to\ the\ drug}{Total\ number\ of\ patients} = \frac{1285}{1473} \approx 0.87$$

As a general rule, the odds ratio in favor of an event occurring is calculated as

$$Odds\ ratio = \frac{p(y)}{p(y')} = \frac{p(y)}{1 - p(y)} \tag{7.12}$$

where $p(y)$ is the probability of the event occurring and $p(y')$ is the probability of the event not occurring. Now, assume we try to translate this probability into an equation similar to what we had used for linear regression:

$$p(y) = \alpha + \beta_1 x_1 + \beta_2 x_2 + \cdots + \beta_k x_k \tag{7.13}$$

The result of this equation, $p(y)$ can range between $-\infty$ and $+\infty$, which we know cannot be true as the probability of an event ranges between 0 and 1. In order to both limit the results between 0 and 1 and factor in different features, we can transform this equation from linear into logarithmic. The transforming function is called the "logit function" or "log-odds function" as it is the natural logarithm (*ln*) of the odds ratio [4]:

$$\ln(odds\ ratio) = \ln\left(\frac{p(y)}{1-p(y)}\right) = \alpha + \beta_1 x_1 + \beta_2 x_2 + \cdots + \beta_k x_k \tag{7.14}$$

After simplifying the equation, we will have

$$p(y) = \frac{e^{\alpha+\beta_1 x_1+\beta_2 x_2+\cdots+\beta_k x_k}}{1+e^{\alpha+\beta_1 x_1+\beta_2 x_2+\cdots+\beta_k x_k}} \tag{7.15}$$

This equation, which ranges between 0 and 1, is known as the "sigmoid function" (Fig. 7.7). In order for the result of the equation, $p(y)$, to be 0, the numerator of the equation must be 0. Therefore, we have

$$e^{\alpha+\beta_1 x_1+\beta_2 x_2+\cdots+\beta_k x_k} = 0 \rightarrow \alpha + \beta_1 x_1 + \beta_2 x_2 + \cdots + \beta_k x_k = -\infty \tag{7.16}$$

And for $p(y)$ to be 1, the numerator and the denominator must be equal. Therefore, $e^{\alpha+\beta_1 x_1+\beta_2 x_2+\cdots+\beta_k x_k}$ must approach infinity, meaning

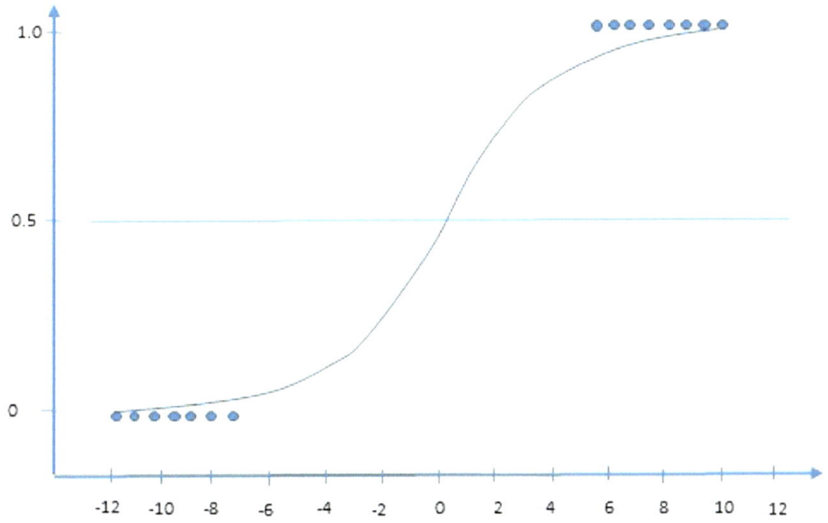

FIGURE 7.7 Sigmoid function representing Eq. (7.15). The output of the function remains in the range of 0 and 1.

that $\alpha + \beta_1 x_1 + \beta_2 x_2 + \cdots + \beta_k x_k$ approaches infinity. This way, even though our coefficients and independent variables can take any value between $-\infty$ and $+\infty$, the estimated probabilities do not fall out of the [0,1] limit. In general, we aim to obtain $Y = 1$ (meaning that the event Y will occur) when $p(y) \geq 0.5$ and $Y = 0$ (meaning that event Y will not occur) if $p(y) < 0.5$. This way, when $\alpha + \beta_1 x_1 + \beta_2 x_2 + \cdots + \beta_k x_k$ is non-negative, $Y = 1$, and when it is negative, $Y = 0$. In fact, the answer (if there is only one independent variable included in our prediction) or a set of answers (in cases where more than one independent variable is included in our model) to the equation $\alpha + \beta_i x_i = 0$ will determine the decision boundary of our model. This decision boundary will be a dot if we make our model based on one independent variable, a line if there are two independent variables, a plane if there are three independent variables, and so on.

What in fact decides to which category a given data point belongs is the probability of that data point belonging to a specific category [4]. Through maximum-likelihood estimation we make sure that with a given set of regression coefficients, the likelihood of each given data point to belong to its actual category is maximum. If for each data point training our model we have a set of features denoted x_i, the observed class denoted y_i, and we let the probability of this data point belonging to class y_i $(y_i = 1)$ be p and the probability of this data point not belonging to class y_i $(y_i = 0)$ be $1 - p$, then the maximum likelihood is calculated as

$$L(\alpha, \beta) = \prod_{i=1}^{N} p(x_i)^{y_i} (1 - p)(x_i)^{1 - y_i} \tag{7.17}$$

This way we can determine the coefficients that determine the importance of each independent variable in classifying the dependent variable. In other words, a maximum-likelihood function helps us choose the set of coefficients that returns the highest probability for getting the observed data among the infinite sets of possible coefficients.

We can associate logistic regression to a Bayesian classifying algorithm if we consider the posterior probability for each class and compare the probabilities. This way, if the probability of belonging to class $y_i = 1$ is greater than the probability of belonging to class $y_i = 0$, then the data point belongs to class $y_i = 1$.

$$P(y_i = 1 | x) = \frac{e^{\alpha + \sum_{i=1}^{n} \beta_i x_i}}{1 + e^{\alpha + \sum_{i=1}^{n} \beta_i x_i}} \tag{7.18}$$

$$P(y_i = 0|x) = \frac{1}{\left(e^{\alpha + \sum_{i=1}^{n} \beta_i x_i}\right)\left(1 + e^{\alpha + \sum_{i=1}^{n} \beta_i x_i}\right)} \tag{7.19}$$

$$P(y_i = 1|x) > P(y_i = 0|x) \Rightarrow \textit{The data point belongs to class } y_i = 1. \tag{7.20}$$

Hands-on logistic regression with R

We start making regression models in R by giving an example of binomial logistic regression using a data set similar to that of Table 7.1. If we categorize neuroblastoma patients into two groups of long-term survival and short-term survival based on whether their survival is above or below 18 months, we will have the data set presented in Table 7.2. In this table, patients with survival time above 18 months are coded as 1 and those with survivals below 18 months are coded as 0. In fact, this way, we have transformed survival from a continuous variable into a discrete binomial variable. In order to make our prediction model, we include all the independent variables. Similar to making a linear regression model, we use the R package "caTools" [10]. The steps of creating a logistic regression model are very similar to those of making a linear regression model. We first import our data and call the necessary packages.

```
> library(caTools)
```

Before attempting to train the model, we need to make sure that our target (dependent) variable is a categorical variable. As mentioned in Chapter 4, categorical variables are presented as "factors" in R. So we need to make sure that our target variable in a logistic regression classification is a factor variable, and if this is not the case, we need to change the class of the variable to a factor variable:

```
> class(table2$Long.term.Survival)
[1] "integer"
> table2$Long.term.Survival=as.factor(table2$Long.term.Survival)
> str(table2)
'data.frame':    36 obs. of  5 variables:
 $ Age               : int  42 2 34 6 32 15 65 23 63 13 ...
 $ Stage             : int  3 1 2 2 2 4 2 4 3 2 ...
 $ Ki67.index....    : int  78 12 46 63 83 80 15 78 51 46 ...
 $ p53               : int  6 0 2 11 23 28 1 13 0 1 ...
 $ Long.term.Survival: Factor w/ 2 levels "0","1": 1 2 2 1 1 1 2 1 2 1 ...
```

TABLE 7.2 Imaginary data on survival of neuroblastoma patients.

Age	Stage	Ki67 index (%)	p53	Long-term survival
42	3	78	6	0
2	1	12	0	1
34	2	46	2	1
6	2	63	11	0
32	2	83	23	0
15	4	80	28	0
65	2	15	1	1
23	4	78	13	0
63	3	51	0	1
13	2	46	1	0
19	1	27	4	1
54	2	58	11	1
72	4	39	13	0
3	3	71	26	0
14	3	62	21	0
56	2	18	1	1
2	1	45	4	1
43	4	58	23	0
16	2	14	1	1
17	3	71	12	0
52	2	64	5	1
17	2	23	0	1
26	2	89	0	0
53	1	23	14	1
1	1	10	0	1
52	1	6	0	1
71	3	41	2	0
4	4	78	21	0

(*Continued*)

TABLE 7.2 (Continued)

Age	Stage	Ki67 index (%)	p53	Long-term survival
15	2	23	11	1
67	1	15	4	0
3	3	64	19	0
46	3	48	3	0
17	2	23	0	1
65	4	61	19	0
37	1	11	0	1
12	3	39	12	0

NOTE...

One thing to remember about making any regression model is that we must make sure our variables are represented in the data set as we mean them to by checking their type using the R built-in function "class." The independent variables included in making a regression model can be either numeric or categorical. In the data sets we import to R, we can either code categorical variables manually, like we did for the data in Table 7.2, or we can leave them as categorical and let R code them on its own. However, if we decide to transform them manually, we must make sure that they are being treated as factor variables, and if their class is "integer," we need to transform them into "factor" variables:

```
> numeric_variable=as.factor(numeric_variable)
```

We can now randomly divide our data set into training and testing subsets similar to the step performed for linear regression:

```
> set.seed(123)
> subsets <- sample(2, nrow(table2), prob=c(0.7, 0.3), replace=T)
> train2 <- table2[subsets==1,]
> test2 <- table2[subsets==2,]
```

Now that we have our training and testing subsets, we should make the logistic regression model based on our independent variables:

```
> binomial <- glm(Long.term.survival~., data=train2,
family="binomial")

> summary(binomial)


Call:

glm(formula = Long.term.survival ~ ., family = "binomial", data =
train2)


Deviance Residuals:

    Min        1Q    Median        3Q       Max

-1.9850   -0.4656   -0.1198    0.5762    1.7398


Coefficients:

               Estimate Std. Error z value Pr(>|z|)

(Intercept)     4.46869    2.07359   2.155   0.0312 *

Age            -0.01337    0.02840  -0.471   0.6378

Stage          -0.67612    1.03217  -0.655   0.5124

Ki67.index.... -0.04167    0.03022  -1.379   0.1680

p53            -0.11295    0.11560  -0.977   0.3285

---

Signif. codes:  0 '***' 0.001 '**' 0.01 '*' 0.05 '.' 0.1 ' ' 1


(Dispersion parameter for binomial family taken to be 1)


    Null deviance: 31.841  on 22  degrees of freedom

Residual deviance: 18.117  on 18  degrees of freedom

AIC: 28.117


Number of Fisher Scoring iterations: 5
```

Significance of coefficients is outlined: Of the variables included, only the stage of the disease helps determine the category of the patients. Two other parameters in the output that indicate the efficacy of the model are the "Null deviance" and "Residual deviance." These parameters indicate the goodness-of-fit for our model and are similar to R-squared in linear regression. However, unlike R-squared, lower values of deviance indicate a better performance of the model. But what is the difference between the null deviance and residual deviance? We have explained the mean model earlier in this chapter—a model that includes no independent variable and only factors in the intercept when making the model. Null deviance represents the goodness-of-fit for the mean model. The residual deviance is the goodness-of-fit for a model that is made based on intercepts and independent variable(s). On the contrary, we assume that there is a model that includes the parameters of all data points when creating the model. Such a model is called a saturated model, and the values it predicts for each data point is equal to their actual value. The performance of the model we create is ideally in between the mean model and the saturated model with outcomes closer to the saturated model than the mean model. If the residual deviance is smaller than the null deviance, it can be concluded that our model has better performance over the mean model. In our model, including four independent variables, as is reflected on the degree of freedom, led to a noteworthy reduction in deviance from 31.841 for null deviance to 18.117 for residual deviance, which shows that the inclusion of independent variables improves the performance of the model in general. Another parameter in the output of our model is AIC (Akaike information criterion), which similar to R-squared lets us know when the inclusion of the independent variables does not improve the performance of our model. AIC can serve as a comparative parameter when we want to compare different regression models based on the same data set. In this case, the model with the smallest AIC is the preferred model. Another parameter that can be seen in the summary of our regression model is the number of Fisher Scoring iterations. This parameter indicates the number of times a maximum-likelihood algorithm was used to fit our model [4,13].

Now that we have trained our model, it is time to see how well our model classifies our testing subset and, as a result, the unseen data.

```
> prediction=predict(binomial, test2, type="response")
> prediction
         2          4          5          8         11         16
20         21
0.96323655 0.30333770 0.03331554 0.03690153 0.87671429 0.81829443
0.10900613 0.30781775
        24         26         31         32         34
0.63281989 0.94518517 0.08220566 0.37434536 0.02203876
```

As can be noted, the predictions are returned in the format of probabilities between 0 and 1. Now we need to determine the cutoff for classification so that these probabilities will be translated into a category of each data point. Here we set the classification cutoff to 0.5.

```
> ConfusionMatrix=table(Actual=test2$Long.term.survival,
Predicted=ifelse(prediction> 0.5, 1, 0))

> ConfusionMatrix

       Predicted

Actual 0 1

     0 7 0

     1 1 5
```

Confusion matrices were discussed in Chapter 5 as a means of assessing the accuracy of classification models. The numbers on the diagonal of the matrix indicate the number of data points that have been correctly classified, and what is not on the diagonal is the number of data points misclassified. Therefore, in order to assess the accuracy of our model, we need to divide the number of correctly classified cases by the total number of cases:

$$Model' saccuracy = \frac{number\ of\ cases\ correctly\ classified}{total\ number\ of\ cases} = \frac{7+5}{7+5+1} \approx 0.92$$

This means that our model predicts the survival class of a given case 92% of the times if we know patient's age, neuroblastoma stage, Ki-67 index, and p53 expression level.

Multinomial logistic regression

We learned how maximum-likelihood algorithms help us create logistic regression models that classify binomial variables. But as mentioned earlier in the chapter, logistic regression models also do an amazing job in classifying categorical variables into more than two classes, say, k classes. However, there are some differences between the binomial logistic regression and the multinomial logistic regression. In binomial logistic regression, we set the cutoff for probabilities based on our purposes and the model makes decisions based on that cutoff value. However, in multinomial regression, as we have more than two categories, the decision that to which category an observation belongs depends on the ratio of the possibilities. The category with the highest probability will be chosen as the category of that specific observation. Another difference is that unlike binomial logistic regression in which we had to set the occurrence of the event to 1, in the case of multinomial logistic regression, we can arbitrarily assign 1, . . ., k to each of the k possible outcomes. We skip the mathematics behind the multinomial regression as it is to some extent similar to that of the binomial logistic regression.

Hands-on multinomial logistic regression in R

In order to make the comparison of the methods and results easier, we use the same data set as presented in Table 7.1, with the only exception that instead of categorizing survival of patients into long- and short-term for patients surviving above or below 18 months, we classify patients into three groups of short-, intermediate-, and long-term survival for those surviving below 12 months, between 12 months and 24 months, and above 24 months, respectively. This data set is similar to the data set used in training Naïve Bayes classifier in Chapter 6.

Let us import our data set, which is presented in Table 7.3 (data). Note that unlike the data in Table 7.2, we have not transformed survival of patients into numeric codes beforehand. Similar to what was observed with the logistic regression, the target variable is not considered a factor variable, and we need to transform it into a factor variable. This will automatically assign 1 to the first class appearing among the independent variables, 2 to the second non-iterated class, and so on.

TABLE 7.3 Imaginary data on survival of neuroblastoma patients.

Age	Stage	Ki67 index (%)	p53	Survival
42	3	78	6	Intermediate
2	1	12	0	Long
34	2	46	2	Long
6	2	63	11	Long
32	2	83	23	Short
15	4	80	28	Short
65	2	15	1	Long
23	4	78	13	Intermediate
63	3	51	0	Long

(Continued)

TABLE 7.3 (Continued)

Age	Stage	Ki67 index (%)	p53	Survival
13	2	46	1	Intermediate
19	1	27	4	Long
54	2	58	11	Long
72	4	39	13	Intermediate
3	3	71	26	Short
14	3	62	21	Intermediate
56	2	18	1	Long
2	1	45	4	Long
43	4	58	23	Short
16	2	14	1	Long
17	3	71	12	Intermediate
52	2	64	5	Long
17	2	23	0	Long
26	2	89	0	Short
53	1	23	14	Long
1	1	10	0	Long
52	1	6	0	Long
71	3	41	2	Intermediate
4	4	78	21	Short
15	2	23	11	Long
67	1	15	4	Long
3	3	64	19	Short
46	3	48	3	Intermediate
17	2	23	0	Long
65	4	61	19	Long
37	1	11	0	Long
12	3	39	12	Short

```
> str(table3)
'data.frame':   36 obs. of  5 variables:
 $ Age           : int  42 2 34 6 32 15 65 23 63 13 ...
 $ Stage         : int  3 1 2 2 2 4 2 4 3 2 ...
 $ Ki67.index....: int  78 12 46 63 83 80 15 78 51 46 ...
 $ p53           : int  6 0 2 11 23 28 1 13 0 1 ...
 $ Survival      : chr  "Intermediate" "Long" "Long" "Long" ...
> table3$Survival <- as.factor(table3$Survival)
> table3$Stage <- as.factor(table3$Stage)
> str(table3)
'data.frame':   36 obs. of  5 variables:
 $ Age           : int  42 2 34 6 32 15 65 23 63 13 ...
 $ Stage         : Factor w/ 4 levels "1","2","3","4": 3 1 2 2 2 4 2 4
3 2 ...
 $ Ki67.index....: int  78 12 46 63 83 80 15 78 51 46 ...
 $ p53           : int  6 0 2 11 23 28 1 13 0 1 ...
 $ Survival      : Factor w/ 3 levels "Intermediate",..: 1 2 2 2 3 3 2
1 2 1 ...
```

We can now divide our data set into training and testing subsets, and train the model using the multinomial() function from the "nnet" package [14]:

```
> library(nnet)
> set.seed(123)
> subsets <- sample(2, nrow(table3), prob=c(0.7, 0.3), replace=T)
> train3 <- table3[subsets==1,]
> test3 <- table3[subsets==2,]
> Model3=multinom(Survival~., data=train3)
# weights:  24 (14 variable)
initial  value 25.268083
iter  10 value 10.181354
iter  20 value 5.803616
iter  30 value 4.278391
iter  40 value 4.079925
iter  50 value 3.722844
iter  60 value 3.696492
iter  70 value 3.687783
iter  80 value 3.667251
iter  90 value 3.596202
iter 100 value 3.587148
final  value 3.587148
stopped after 100 iterations
```

We can see that the model had an initial error value of approximately 25.26, and after 100 iterations, this value was significantly reduced to ~3.58. We investigate other aspects of the model now:

```
> summary(Model3)
Call:
multinom(formula = Survival ~ ., data = train3)


Coefficients:
      (Intercept)        Age     Stage2    Stage3    Stage4
Ki67.index....          p53
Long    49.346074  0.1063328 -46.46649 -52.10090 -87.45311    -
0.09539708 -0.009238947
Short    7.876121 -2.3905139 -30.15958  28.11424 121.16286
1.01408402 -3.405561048


Std. Errors:
      (Intercept)       Age     Stage2    Stage3        Stage4
Ki67.index....       p53
Long     3.462717 0.1153840  2.062863  4.290952 2.922020e-12
0.09442392 0.3165017
Short   47.166401 0.8912456 24.286657 16.215989 1.508572e+01
0.92193529 1.3633623


Residual Deviance: 7.174296
AIC: 35.1743
```

As we could see in the mathematics behind logistic regressions, we choose one of the k categories of the dependent variable as a reference, and the probabilities of belonging to other categories will be weighed against the probability of belonging to the reference level, what we know as the odds ratio. We can determine which of the k categories we wish to set as the reference level; however, if we do not choose the reference level, the category set to 1 will automatically be chosen as the reference level. This is reflected in the summary of the model as the coefficients and standard errors are only reported for the other two categories.

As is the case for binomial logistic regression, a lower residual deviance and AIC indicate a better goodness-of-fit for our model.

However, it is still too early to judge our model as we need to first see how well it performs when tested on unseen data, which in this case is our testing subset.

We test the performance of our model by observing how accurate it is in classifying a testing subset. Before determining the class of each observation testing subset, let us see the probabilities of belonging to each of the three categories of the dependent variable:

```
> predicted_probabilities=predict(Model3, test3, type="probs")
> predicted_probabilities
   Intermediate         Long        Short
2  9.420590e-22 1.000000e+00 4.010450e-15
4  9.304463e-01 6.951918e-02 3.457025e-05
5  8.639176e-01 1.360824e-01 3.746680e-41
8  5.158609e-48 8.734861e-67 1.000000e+00
11 6.706999e-22 1.000000e+00 3.137363e-32
16 8.179936e-04 9.991820e-01 3.508124e-65
20 3.146103e-12 1.249431e-15 1.000000e+00
21 9.472292e-02 9.052771e-01 1.271666e-44
24 1.351509e-23 1.000000e+00 8.926659e-86
26 2.609201e-24 1.000000e+00 3.117491e-72
31 2.506957e-13 4.106726e-17 1.000000e+00
32 9.220331e-01 7.796694e-02 3.477302e-16
34 1.000000e+00 7.055309e-17 2.101484e-13
```

For each observation, the category with the highest probability is chosen as the category of the observation:

```
> predicted_category=predict(Model3, test3)
> predicted_category
 [1] Long         Intermediate Intermediate Short        Long
Long
 [7] Short        Long         Long         Long         Short
Intermediate
[13] Intermediate
Levels: Intermediate Long Short
```

We can now determine the performance of our model by getting the confusion matrix of the model:

```
> confusion_matrix=table(predicted_category,test3$Survival)
> confusion_matrix

predicted_category Intermediate Long Short
      Intermediate            1    2     1
      Long                    0    6     0
      Short                   2    0     1
```

$$Model'saccuracy = \frac{number\ of\ cases\ correctly\ classified}{total\ number\ of\ cases} = \frac{1+6+1}{1+6+1+2+2+1} \approx 0.61$$

Even though our model correctly classifies observations in more than 50% of cases, the accuracy of the model is not reliable since if we make the confusion matric using the caret package similar to the previous chapter, the *P*-value for accuracy compared to no information rate is above 0.05. We can improve it either by changing the independent variables upon which the model is trained or by changing the algorithm based on which we build the model. Other classifying algorithms will be introduced in future chapters, which can be helpful in improving predictive models' performance.

References

[1] F. Galton, Regression towards mediocrity in hereditary stature, The Journal of the Anthropological Institute of Great Britain and Ireland 15 (1886) 246–263.
[2] A. Schneider, G. Hommel, M. Blettner, Linear regression analysis: part 14 of a series on evaluation of scientific publications, Deutsches Arzteblatt International 107 (44) (2010) 776–782.
[3] M.J. Hayat, M. Higgins, Understanding poisson regression, The Journal of Nursing Education 53 (4) (2014) 207–215.
[4] V. Bewick, L. Cheek, J. Ball, Statistics review 14: logistic regression, Critical Care (London, England) 9 (1) (2005) 112–118.
[5] S. Liu, M. Lu, H. Li, Y. Zuo, Prediction of gene expression patterns with generalized linear regression model, Frontiers in Genetics 10 (2019) 120.
[6] K. Godfrey, Simple linear regression in medical research, The New England Journal of Medicine 313 (26) (1985) 1629–1636.
[7] A. Heath, N. Kunst, C. Jackson, M. Strong, F. Alarid-Escudero, J.D. Goldhaber-Fiebert, et al., Calculating the expected value of sample information in practice: considerations from 3 case studies, Medical Decision Making: An International Journal of the Society for Medical Decision Making 40 (3) (2020) 314–326.
[8] J. Lever, M. Krzywinski, N. Altman, Model selection and overfitting, Nature Methods 13 (2016) 703–704.

[9] W. Revelle, Psych: Procedures for Psychological, Psychometric, and Personality Research. Northwestern University, Evanston, IL. R package version 2.1.6, 2021. https://CRAN.R-project.org/package = psych.
[10] J. Tuszynski, caTools. R package version 1.17, 2014.
[11] A. Colin Cameron, F. Windmeijer, An R-squared measure of goodness of fit for some common nonlinear regression models, Journal of Econometrics 77 (2) (1997) 329–342.
[12] U. Grömping, Relative importance for linear regression in R: the package relaimpo, Journal of Statistical Software 17 (1) (2006) 1–27.
[13] S. Sperandei, Understanding logistic regression analysis, Biochemia Medica 24 (1) (2014) 12–18.
[14] W.N. Venables, B.D. Ripley, Modern Applied Statistics with S, fourth ed., Springer, New York, 2002ISBN 0-387-95457-0. Available from: https://www.stats.ox.ac.uk/pub/MASS4/.

CHAPTER

8

Linear and quadratic discriminant analysis in R

Discriminant-based classifiers

Thus far, we learned about some regression and classification algorithms. In this chapter, we will learn two other classification algorithms: linear discriminant analysis (LDA) and quadratic discriminant analysis (QDA). In Chapter 5, we became familiar with the concept of defining borders that could categorize data points into two or more groups. The simplest form of such borders being a straight line is the idea behind LDA [1] for which we will study the principles in this chapter. However, we also learned that this simple form of border may not result in high levels of accuracy, but as there is a tradeoff between accuracy and predictability, LDA is still a popular method of classification, even though it is mostly recognized as a method for dimension reduction.

Simplicity of discriminant analysis-based methods makes them among the favorite classification algorithms. However, as always, the choice of the algorithm depends mostly on the type of data set we have in hand. Even though logistic regression and Bayes classifiers that were described in previous chapters are powerful tools for classifying categorical data, like other algorithms they also come with their own set of assumptions that limit their use for some data sets. For example, we learned that logistic regression is a powerful algorithm for classification, especially if we have categorical independent variables and binary dependent variables. But as we add to our machine learning skills, we learn that there might be better algorithms for the classification of categorical data sets with more than two classes in the dependent variable. Two of such algorithms are LDA and QDA.

Immunoinformatics of Cancers
DOI: https://doi.org/10.1016/B978-0-12-822400-7.00009-9

Imagine a small data set of five numeric independent variables and a dependent variable with four classes. We have several options to build a classification model based on this data set that we must weight against one another. For an instance, even though logistic regression is powerful classification algorithm and does not set limits for the type of the independent variables, it may not be the best algorithm for the classification of the described data set as the dependent variable in this data set is multinomial. As mentioned, LDA and QDA can be used for multinomial classifications; however, they have their own set of assumptions that must be met for these classifiers to perform their best.

Discriminant analysis-based classifiers assume that the dependent variable is categorical, and that each class in the dependent variable constitutes a roughly equal portion of the dependent variable. Therefore, discrepancies in proportions of classes in the data set can impair their performance. Another assumption is that the independent variables are not correlated and are drawn from a multivariate normal distribution. Even though it is rare for real-world data sets to conform to the assumption regarding independence of variables, specifically in data sets generated in life sciences, discriminant analysis can still be used in such data sets as they have some level of robustness to nonconformity to their assumptions. One of the most important assumptions of LDA and QDA is that they assume each independent variable to be normally distributed for each of the classes in the dependent variable. But what determines the choice between QDA and LDA is the homogeneity of variance in independent variables for each class of the dependent variable. LDA assumes that covariances among independent variables are equal for each class of the dependent variable, while QDA does not set any such limitation.

Even though discriminant analysis-based algorithms set more limitations compared to logistic regression, there are instances where they are preferred over other classification algorithms. One such instance is when the sample size is small and the data meet the assumption of the discriminant-analysis-based algorithms: LDA and QDA perform a steadier job compared to the logistic regression. But how do these models classify data? Let us take a glance at the mathematics behind each of these algorithms. Remember, if you are not a fan of mathematics, you can head straight to the hands-on LDA and QDA in R.

Linear discriminant analysis

We mentioned that LDA is similar to logistic regression in that it is used for classification purposes. But the way LDA performs classifications is similar to linear regression in many aspects. Similar to multiple regression, in discriminant analysis we plot each independent variable against the dependent variable to find the most appropriate independent variables to build our model upon. Then LDA creates linear equations to explain the data set. In fact, LDA finds a linear combination of the independent variables to classify observations in the dependent variable most efficiently.

But how does LDA decide to which category of the dependent variable a data point belongs? It classifies data points by trying to categorize data sets into groups whose centers have the maximum possible distance from one another, and in the meantime have the least intragroup variance [2]. In simple words, it tries to place all similar data points in one category (least intragroup variance) in a way that these categories are easily distinguishable from one another (maximum distance between the centers). In fact, what helps LDA make the decision is the difference between mean (μ) and variance (σ^2) of different categories. It is expected that the more the difference (or the distance) between the averages (centers) of groups is, and the less scattered data points around that center are, the easier it will be to classify data points into these groups (Fig. 8.1).

For a data set with K classes in the dependent variable, each class has a prior probability of π_k so that $\pi_1 + \pi_2 + \ldots + \pi_k = 1$. From Bayes' rule, the posterior probability of these classes is:

$$\Pr(C = k|X = x) = \frac{f_k(x)\pi_k}{\sum_{i=1}^{k} f_i(x)\pi_i}, \tag{8.1}$$

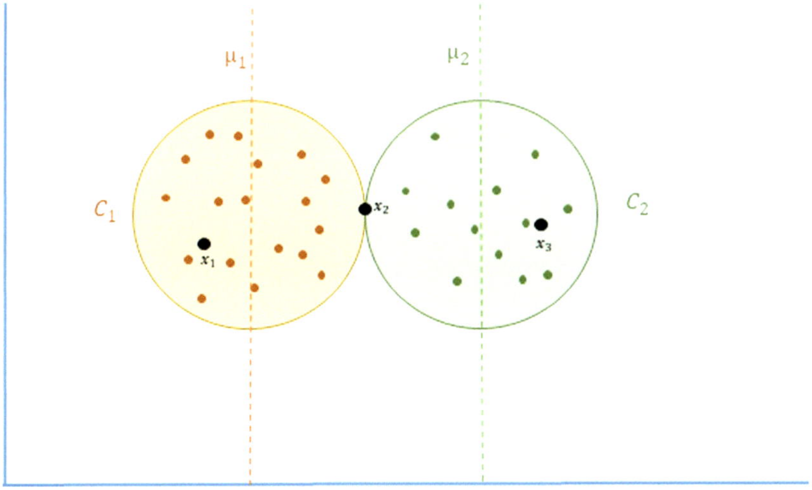

FIGURE 8.1 Schematic representation of a data set with two categories for the dependent variable. We aim to classify x_1, x_2, and x_3 into either of C_1 and C_2 categories.

where $f_k(x)$ is the density function of X condition with K classes. The maximum-a-posteriori for each class will be:

$$C(x) = \arg max_k \Pr(C = k|X = x) = \arg max_k f_k(x)\pi_k \tag{8.2}$$

Given that LDA assumes a Gaussian distribution for the density, the following equation holds:

$$f_k(x) = |2\pi\Sigma_k|^{-1/2} \exp\left(-\frac{1}{2}(x-\mu_k)^T\Sigma_k^{-1}(x-\mu_k)\right) \tag{8.3}$$

where $|\Sigma_k|$ is the determinant for covariance matrix for class K and μ_k is the mean for class K. As LDA assumes equal covariance matrices for different classes, the following equation holds:

$$C(x) = \arg max_k x^T\Sigma^{-1}\mu_k - \frac{1}{2}\mu_k^T\Sigma^{-1}\mu_k + log\pi_k = \arg max_k \delta_k(x), \tag{8.4}$$

where $\delta_k(x)$ is the discriminant function for class K. By calculating the covariance matrix, mean, and prior probability based on the data set in hand, we can find the probability of a data point being assigned to any of the classes in the dependent variable.

In QDA, however, as each class of dependent variable has its specific covariance matrix, we need to estimate this for each of the K classes. Therefore, the discriminant function for QDA will be as follows:

$$\delta_k(x) = -\frac{1}{2}\log|\Sigma_k| - \frac{1}{2}(x-\mu_k)^T\Sigma_k^{-1}(x-\mu_k) + log\pi_k \tag{8.5}$$

Now let us see how these probabilities are estimated in practice:

Hands-on linear discriminant analysis in R

As mentioned earlier, LDA can perform better in instances of multinomial classification when compared to logistic regression algorithm [3]. However, before applying discriminant analysis to create a predictive model based on our data set, we need to test the homogeneity of variances in independent variables for each subcategory of the dependent variable. A number of tests are available for this evaluation including Bartlett's test, Levene's test, and Fligner-Killeen's test [4]. In this chapter, we choose to evaluate whether variances in different classes of the dependent variable have homogeneous variances or not by using Levene's test in R, because compared to Bartlett's test, it is less sensitive to deviation from normality. If the results are supportive of this homogeneity, we must choose LDA over QDA, otherwise, QDA performs a better job at classification. However, for learning purposes, we use both LDA and QDA to create the predictive model and to compare their results.

In order to compare the performance of different classification models, we use the same data set that was used in Table 6.2 to train both LDA and QDA classifiers. Of course, as assumptions for LDA are stricter than those for QDA, deviations from these assumptions are more probable to affect the performance of LDA than that of QDA. As many real-world data do not conform to the assumptions of machine learning algorithms, we try to reflect that in our example data set.

Before evaluating the homogeneity of variances, we need to ensure that the structure of the data set is as it is supposed to be. The stage of the disease and survival of patients are categorical variables. So, we need to change the class of these variables to factor:

```
> str(data)
'data.frame':     36 obs. of  5 variables:
 $ Age          : int  42 2 34 6 32 15 65 23 63 13 ...
 $ Stage        : int  3 1 2 2 2 4 2 4 3 2 ...
 $ Ki67.index....: int  78 12 46 63 83 80 15 78 51 46 ...
 $ p53          : int  6 0 2 11 23 28 1 13 0 1 ...
 $ Survival     : chr  "Intermediate" "Long" "Long" "Long" ...
```

We need to modify the class of the "Stage" and "Survival" variables to factor variables:

```
> data$Stage <- as.factor(data$Stage)
> data$Survival <- as.factor(data$Survival)
```

In order to test homogeneity of variances in continuous variables, we use the leveneTest() function to form the "car" package [5]:

```
> install.packages("car")
> library(car)
> leveneTest(data$Age, data$Survival, center=mean)
Levene's Test for Homogeneity of Variance (center = mean)
      Df F value Pr(>F)
group  2   2.993 0.0639 .
      33
---
Signif. codes:  0 '***' 0.001 '**' 0.01 '*' 0.05 '.' 0.1 ' ' 1
> leveneTest(data$Ki67.index...., data$Survival, center=mean)
Levene's Test for Homogeneity of Variance (center = mean)
      Df F value Pr(>F)
group  2   1.182 0.3193
      33
> leveneTest(data$p53, data$Survival, center=mean)
Levene's Test for Homogeneity of Variance (center = mean)
      Df F value Pr(>F)
group  2  0.8918 0.4196
      33
```

As the *P*-values for all the three independent variables are above the alpha of 0.05 (0.0639, 0.3193, and 0.4196 for Age, Ki67 index, and p53, respectively), the variances of samples in the three independent variables for each class of short, intermediate, and long survival is homogeneous. Therefore, we can use LDA to create our classification model. But before creating our model, let us see how our data points are distributed among the different independent variables. For this purpose, we use the pairs.panels() function from the "psych" package [6] (Fig. 8.2).

```
> library(psych)
pairs.panels(data[1:5],bg=c("red","yellow","blue")[data $Survival],
            pch=21,)
```

Fig. 8.2 shows the resulting scatterplot. As can be seen, data points can be roughly categorized into different classes through visual inspection. Based on this figure, data do not follow a normal distribution; however, their deviation from normal distribution can be negligible due to the robustness of LDA in tolerating slight deviations from its assumptions. However, a thorough look at the data shows that there is substantial difference in the nature of the numerical variables in that they have different

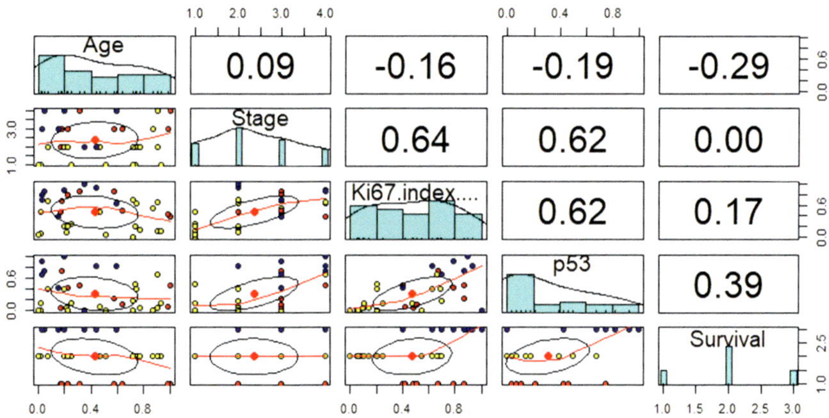

FIGURE 8.2 Scatterplot showing the distribution of data points among different independent variables along with the correlation of the variables. Data in each variable are normally distributed.

scales and ranges which can affect their impact on classification models if left unchanged. Therefore, we need to make sure that these variables are normalized before using them to build our model.

As mentioned earlier, the main aspect of the variables that need to be taken care of during normalization is the discrepancies in their ranges. Therefore, we normalize continuous independent variables for their ranges using the preProcess() function from the "caret" package [7]:

```
> library(caret)
> preprocessParams <- preProcess(data[,1:4], method=c("range"))
> preprocessParams
Created from 36 samples and 4 variables

Pre-processing:
  - ignored (1)
  - re-scaling to [0, 1] (3)
```

We transformed all continuous variables using the preprocess() function, which automatically ignores categorical variables. As the output of the function shows, it has re-scaled all variables between 0 and 1:

```
> transformed <- predict(preprocessParams, data[,1:5])
> head(transformed)
         Age Stage Ki67.index....        p53     Survival
1 0.57746479     3     0.86746988 0.21428571 Intermediate
2 0.01408451     1     0.07228916 0.00000000         Long
3 0.46478873     2     0.48192771 0.07142857         Long
4 0.07042254     2     0.68674699 0.39285714         Long
5 0.43661972     2     0.92771084 0.82142857        Short
6 0.19718310     4     0.89156627 1.00000000        Short
```

We can now divide this transformed data into training and testing subsets:

```
> data <- transformed
> set.seed(123)
> subsets <- sample(2, nrow(data), prob=c(0.7, 0.3), replace=T)
> train <- data[subsets==1,]
> test <- data[subsets==2,]
```

Now our data are ready to train the LDA and QDA models. For this purpose, we use "MASS" package [8]. We start off by creating our LDA model.

```
> install.packages("MASS")

> library(MASS)

> LDA <- lda(Survival~., data=train)

> LDA
Call:
lda(Survival ~ ., data = train)

Prior probabilities of groups:
Intermediate         Long        Short
   0.2173913    0.5217391    0.2608696

Group means:
                   Age    Stage2     Stage3 Stage4 Ki67.index....       p53
Intermediate 0.5830986 0.2000000 0.60000000    0.2      0.5686747 0.3071429
Long         0.4413146 0.5833333 0.08333333    0.0      0.2630522 0.1011905
Short        0.2276995 0.1666667 0.33333333    0.5      0.7610442 0.6547619

Coefficients of linear discriminants:
                      LD1        LD2
Age             1.1755178 -1.2096959
Stage2         -0.3006302 -0.4498758
Stage3         -1.9200931 -2.5440588
Stage4         -2.9009423 -1.6415160
Ki67.index.... -2.8928270  0.2091053
p53            -0.1472585  2.2514280

Proportion of trace:
   LD1    LD2
0.8968 0.1032
```

Prior probabilities in the model show the proportion of each class in the dependent variable. Based on what we learned in the Bayes theory, prior probability will have a large impact on the classifications. Group means give us an idea of how close or how far classes of dependent variable are based on each independent variable. Similar to linear regression, coefficients show the importance of each independent variable in making predictions, here for the class of the dependent variable. The number of linear discriminant functions depends on the number of classes in the dependent variables. For a data set with K classes in the dependent variable, LDA models will return K-1 linear discriminant functions as LD1, LD2, ..., LD

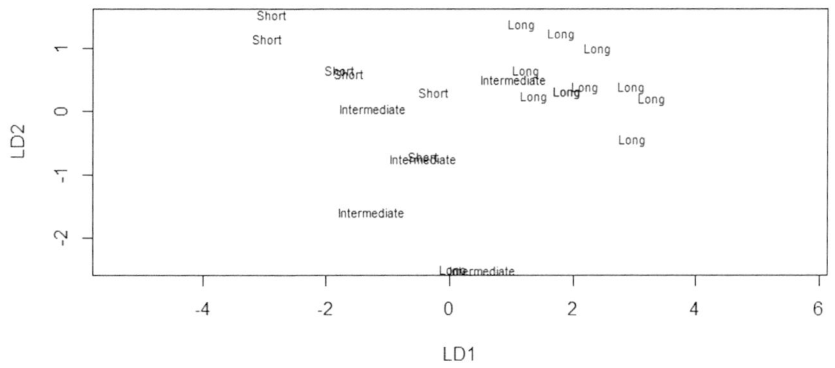

FIGURE 8.3 Linear discriminant analysis plot showing how the two discriminant functions can classify the data points.

(K-1). Therefore, here we have two linear discriminant functions. Based on the proportions of each discriminant function, it is shown that LD1 has a much better performance in explaining the data set compared to LD2. However, there is no single discriminant function that can explain the entire data set, and all discriminant functions are required to explain 100% of the data set (LD1 + LD2 + . . . + LD (K-1) = 1).

In order to visualize how these discriminant functions can be used to classify the data points, we plot the model (Fig. 8.3):

```
> plot(LDA)
```

Classification of LDA based on LD1 and LD2 shows a good classification of observations; however, there are some instances where classes of observations overlap, hence affecting a model's performance. On the other hand, we must remember that these classifications are being performed on the training model. We can only rely on the accuracy of our model by implementing it to classify data points in the testing subset:

```
> predict_LDA <- predict(LDA, test)
> predict_LDA
$class
 [1] Long        Long        Short       Short       Long        Long
 [7] Short       Long        Long        Long        Short
Intermediate
[13] Short
```

```
Levels: Intermediate Long Short

$posterior
   Intermediate         Long        Short
2  0.0036303349 0.9961315453 2.381198e-04
4  0.1207873025 0.5998538893 2.793588e-01
5  0.0719360727 0.3267392908 6.013246e-01
8  0.0525548605 0.0001161332 9.473290e-01
11 0.0059733834 0.9934048129 6.218036e-04
16 0.0064940026 0.9934663122 3.968512e-05
20 0.4895082301 0.0048095100 5.056823e-01
21 0.1316492761 0.8512373224 1.711340e-02
24 0.0011285860 0.9988056638 6.575018e-05
26 0.0009724097 0.9990232384 4.351838e-06
31 0.2292809174 0.0051094438 7.656096e-01
32 0.9341635379 0.0415041361 2.433233e-02
34 0.3150156056 0.0081675189 6.768169e-01

$x
          LD1         LD2
2   1.8127136  0.87717957
4  -0.2570620  1.37212782
5  -0.5867682  1.94442511
8  -3.1092305  0.08944855
11  1.5503387  0.94695676
16  2.1917599 -0.39722246
20 -1.9784883 -0.80890996
21  0.5012431  0.10845168
24  2.2000837  1.16166982
26  2.8496631  0.01016501
31 -2.0031218 -0.02515677
32 -0.6493874 -2.08462922
34 -1.8529025 -0.18652616
```

There are three components in the results of applying our model to the test data. The first component, class, shows how the model has classified each of the observations in testing subset in the data set. The second component, posterior, shows the probability of each data point belonging to each of the three classes in the dependent variable. Finally, "x" shows the accordance of coordination of each sample with either of the discriminant functions. Therefore, if a sample has approximately equal scores for each of the discriminant functions, the chances of such sample being misclassified might be higher.

In order to understand the efficacy of our classification model, we can create the confusion matrix, similar to other classification models:

```
> ConfusionMatrix_LDA <- confusionMatrix(predict_LDA$class, test$Survival)
> ConfusionMatrix_LDA
Confusion Matrix and Statistics

              Reference
Prediction     Intermediate Long Short
  Intermediate            1    0     0
  Long                    0    7     0
  Short                   2    1     2

Overall Statistics

               Accuracy : 0.7692
                 95% CI : (0.4619, 0.9496)
    No Information Rate : 0.6154
    P-Value [Acc > NIR] : 0.1986

                  Kappa : 0.61

 Mcnemar's Test P-Value : NA

Statistics by Class:

                     Class: Intermediate Class: Long Class: Short
Sensitivity                      0.33333      0.8750       1.0000
Specificity                      1.00000      1.0000       0.7273
Pos Pred Value                   1.00000      1.0000       0.4000
Neg Pred Value                   0.83333      0.8333       1.0000
Prevalence                       0.23077      0.6154       0.1538
Detection Rate                   0.07692      0.5385       0.1538
Detection Prevalence             0.07692      0.5385       0.3846
Balanced Accuracy                0.66667      0.9375       0.8636
```

Based on the confusion matrix, our model has an accuracy of ~77%, which shows an acceptable performance of our model. Another way of evaluating a model's performance is visualizing model classifications.

```
> ldahist(data=predict_LDA$x[,1], g= train$Survival)
> ldahist(data=predict_LDA$x[,2], g= train$Survival)
```

The two histograms in Fig. 8.4 and 8.5 show the performance of LD1 and LD2, respectively, in classifying the data points. Therefore, it is expected that a successful classification function results in minimum overlap between the groups. Based on these histograms, LD1 has better performance due to little overlap between the groups, which is expected due to better coverage of observations in LD1 compared to LD2.

Another method to better visualize the performance of the model, which is basically a clearer visualization of Fig. 8.3, is the scatter plot of predictions. However, note that here we are using the test data rather than the training data. For this purpose, we color-code the

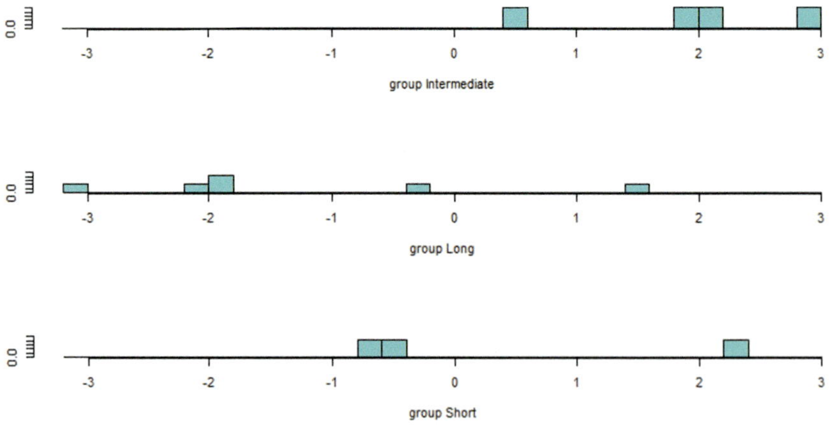

FIGURE 8.4 Histograms showing classifying samples in into short, intermediate, and long groups based on discriminant function LD1. The negligible overlap between the histograms shows high accuracy of the classification function.

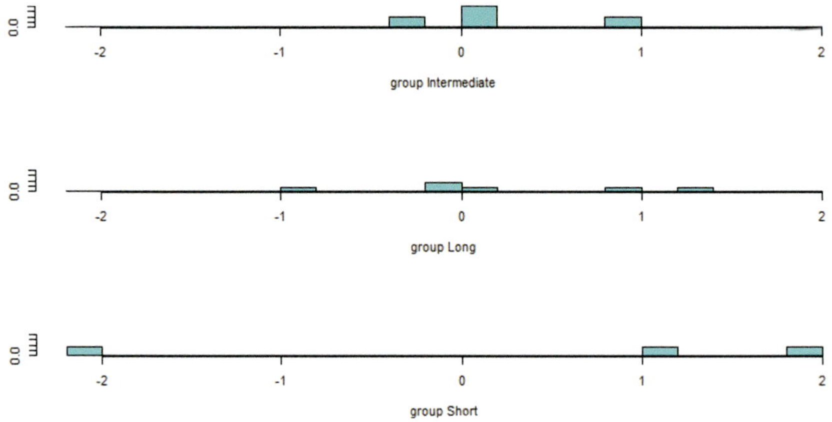

FIGURE 8.5 Histograms showing classifying samples in Table 1 into short, intermediate, and long groups based on the discriminant function LD2. The vertical overlap between histograms shows poor performance of the function.

classes in the samples (Fig. 8.6). For this plot, we use the "ggplot2" package.

```
> library(ggplot2)
> lda.data <- cbind(test$Survival, predict_LDA$x)
> lda.data <- as.data.frame(lda.data)
> ggplot(lda.data, aes(LD1, LD2)) + geom_point(aes(color = test$Survival))
```

Fig. 8.6 shows that the distinction of observation classes is better for the "Long" survival group; however, for the other groups there are

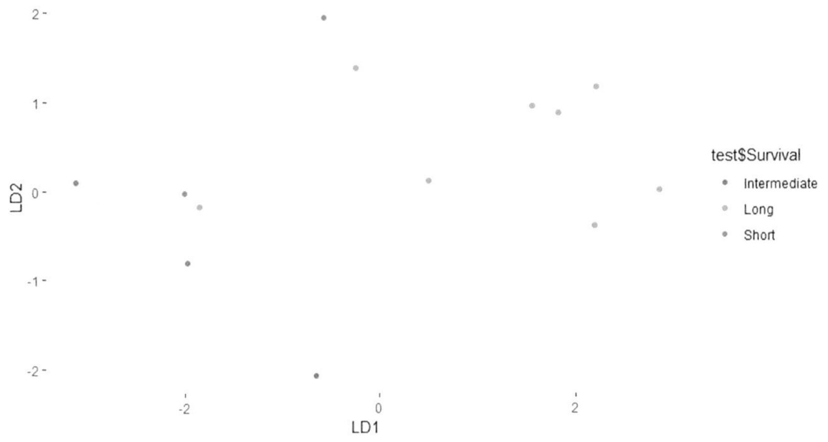

FIGURE 8.6 Scatter plot of the samples and their classes representing the performance of LD1 and LD2 functions.

some overlaps between the observations. There are some limitations in our data that need to be considered when making predictive models. The size of the data set is very small. Furthermore, the proportion of classes in the data are imbalanced. Considering these factors and that assumptions of LDA were not entirely true for our data set, LDA performed relatively well in classifying the data. We now compare the performance of LDA with QDA for the same data set.

Hands-on quadratic discriminant analysis in R

As mentioned throughout the chapter, QDA relaxes the assumption that covariance matrices for all of the classes in the dependent variable are the same. So why do we not always use QDA instead of LDA? One reason is that when the assumption of equality of covariance matrices holds true, LDA performs a better job than QDA. Also, LDA performs a better job for the classification of small data sets. Another advantage of LDA over QDA is that LDA can be used for dimensionality reduction, but QDA cannot. In addition, there are some limitations that using QDA can impose. As an example, in order to train a QDA model, the number of observations for each class of the target variable must be larger than the number of features of the data set. In order to compare the performance of QDA and LDA, let us classify the data set in Table 6.2 using QDA. The steps for creating a QDA model is similar to that of LDA using the MASS package, and similarly we need to use normalized data to train the model. Given that we had split this standardized data for LDA, we use the same training and testing data to create our QDA model.

```
> QDA <- qda(Survival~., data=train)
Error in qda.default(x, grouping, ...) :
  some group is too small for 'qda'
```

As mentioned earlier, one of the limitations of QDA is that the number of observations in each class of the dependent variable must be greater than the number of variables involved in training the model. In our training data, the number of observations in each of the survival classes is as follows:

```
> sum(train$Survival=="Intermediate")
[1] 5
> sum(train$Survival=="Long")
[1] 12
> sum(train$Survival=="Short")
[1] 6
```

In order to create our QDA model, we need to either provide more data to our model, such as increasing the data size, or change the proportion of division of data set into training and testing samples. In addition, we can change the number of variables involved in training the model. We can either use our background knowledge, use feature selection, or randomly exclude one of the variables. Some of the feature selection methods will be discussed in future chapters. In order to find features that potentially affect our predictions the most, we can use coefficients attributed to each of the variables from Fig. 8.2. "p53," "Age," and "Ki 67 index" have the highest absolute value of coefficients. So, we use these variables to train our QDA model.

```
> QDA <- qda(Survival~ Age + p53 + Ki67.index...., data=train)
> QDA
Call:
qda(Survival ~ Age + p53 + Ki67.index...., data = train)


Prior probabilities of groups:
Intermediate         Long        Short
   0.2173913    0.5217391    0.2608696
```

```
Group means:
                   Age       p53 Ki67.index....
Intermediate 0.5830986 0.3071429      0.5686747
Long         0.4413146 0.1011905      0.2630522
Short        0.2276995 0.6547619      0.7610442
```

As expected, the confusion matrix for QDA will be the same as LDA:

```
> ConfusionMatrix_QDA <- confusionMatrix(test$Survival,predict_QDA$class)
> ConfusionMatrix_QDA
Confusion Matrix and Statistics

              Reference
Prediction     Intermediate Long Short
  Intermediate            1    0     2
  Long                    1    6     1
  Short                   0    0     2

Overall Statistics

               Accuracy : 0.6923
                 95% CI : (0.3857, 0.9091)
    No Information Rate : 0.4615
    P-Value [Acc > NIR] : 0.08198

                  Kappa : 0.5048

 Mcnemar's Test P-Value : 0.26146

Statistics by Class:

                     Class: Intermediate Class: Long Class: Short
Sensitivity                      0.50000      1.0000       0.4000
Specificity                      0.81818      0.7143       1.0000
Pos Pred Value                   0.33333      0.7500       1.0000
Neg Pred Value                   0.90000      1.0000       0.7273
Prevalence                       0.15385      0.4615       0.3846
Detection Rate                   0.07692      0.4615       0.1538
Detection Prevalence             0.23077      0.6154       0.1538
Balanced Accuracy                0.65909      0.8571       0.7000
```

The performance of the model has slightly decreased, which can be due to the exclusion of one of the variables. A comparison of the *P*-values of the LDA and QDA in confusion matrix output shows that the *P*-value of the LDA model is further away from the conventional significant cutoff of 0.05. Therefore, accuracy of the QDA model is more reliable than that of the LDA, even though it is lower in percentage.

There are further discriminant-based classifiers that were not discussed in detail; however, these classifiers are easily generated using the MASS package in R. Of these discriminant-based classifiers, mixture discriminant analysis, flexible discriminant analysis, and regularized discriminant analysis can be named. These classifiers are mainly variants of LDA and the main difference between them is in the presumptions which make them suitable for different data sets.

References

[1] A. Tharwat, T. Gaber, A. Ibrahim, A.E. Hassanien, Linear discriminant analysis: a detailed tutorial, AI Communications 30 (2) (2017) 169–190. Available from: https://doi.org/10.3233/AIC-170729.
[2] B. Ghojogh, M. Crowley, Linear and quadratic discriminant analysis: tutorial, 2019. http://arxiv.org/abs/1906.02590 (accessed August 15, 2021).
[3] L.J. King, Discriminant analysis: a review of recent theoretical contributions and applications, Economic Geography 46 (1970) 367. Available from: https://doi.org/10.2307/143150.
[4] Z. Mu, Comparing the statistical tests for homogeneity of variances, Electronic Theses and Dissertations (2006). Paper 2212.
[5] J. Fox, S. Weisberg, An R Companion to Applied Regression, third ed., Sage, Thousand Oaks, CA, 2019.
[6] W. Revelle, Psych: Procedures for Psychological, Psychometric, and Personality Research, Northwestern University, Evanston, IL, 2021. R package version 2.1.9.
[7] M. Kuhn, Caret package, Journal of Statistical Software 28 (5) (2008).
[8] W.N. Venables, B.D. Ripley, Modern Applied Statistics with S, fourth ed., Springer, New York, 2002.

CHAPTER

9

Support vector machines in R

What is support vector machine?

Support vector machines (SVMs) are kernel-based supervised algorithms used for both classification and regression (support vector regression, SVR) purposes [1]. Kernel functions help us calculate the dot product of two vectors in high dimensions. Kernel helps with transforming data points from the input space to feature space with higher dimensions [2]. Similar to the idea described in the previous chapters regarding defining borders to classify data points into different categories, we try to define borders for our classification (SVM classifier). The idea behind SVRs is also similar to that of the linear regression in that it attempts to find the function that will result in minimum residual errors.

In SVM classification, we try to find the border that is furthest from support vectors [1]. Support vectors are the data points that are closest to the classification border and can affect the configuration of this border in a multidimensional space [1]. The dimensions of this border are determined by our data dimension (i.e., the number of features). In a two-dimensional space, the classification border is a line. In a three-dimensional space, the classification space is a plane, and in higher dimensions, this border becomes a hyperplane. In SVM classification, we aim to maximize the distance between the hyperplane and the support vectors; in other words, we try to maximize the margin between the classification boundary (hyperplane) and the data points. In addition to focusing on support vectors, SVM ignores some data points so that the decision boundary is only affected by the support vectors. This will result in minimizing the loss and increasing model accuracy when faced with new data.

Immunoinformatics of Cancers
DOI: https://doi.org/10.1016/B978-0-12-822400-7.00013-0

There are several advantages to SVM that make it one of the most popular and useful classifiers for real-world data in many fields, including bioinformatics. One of these advantages is the high learning ability of the model and fast computations. Another strength point of SVM compared to linear classifiers, such as logistic regression, is its ability to classify saturated or oversaturated data, which happens when the number of features is larger than the sample size. SVMs were originally developed for binary classification; however, they have been extended to classify multiclass data as well. In this chapter, we review the mathematics behind the binary SVM classifier and use SVM for the classification of the survival of neuroblastoma patients from previous chapters. We also use SVR for the prediction of patient survival from the data set in Chapter 7.

Mathematics behind support vector machine

Consider that we have a data set with n data points to train our SVM classifier. Given that our classifier is basically a hyperplane following $w.x + b = 0$, where w is the weight vector and b is the bias. As mentioned earlier, we choose a margin for the hyperplane and try to maximize the margin. In order to have a margin around our hyperplane of $w.x + b = 0$, we use the following decision function to define two additional hyperplanes around our original hyperplane of $w.x + b = 0$ [3]:

$$f(x) = \text{sign}(w.x + b), \text{sign}(x) = \begin{cases} +1 \text{ if } & x > 0 \\ 0 \text{ if } & x = 0 \\ -1 \text{ if } & x < 0 \end{cases} \tag{9.1}$$

This leads to two hyperplanes of $w.x + b = 1$ and $w.x + b = -1$ surrounding the original hyperplane, with a distance of $\frac{1}{\lambda||w||^2}$ from the original hyperplane. Now, we have a margin of $\frac{2}{||w||^2}$ on either side of the classifying hyperplane, which we need to maximize (Fig. 9.1).

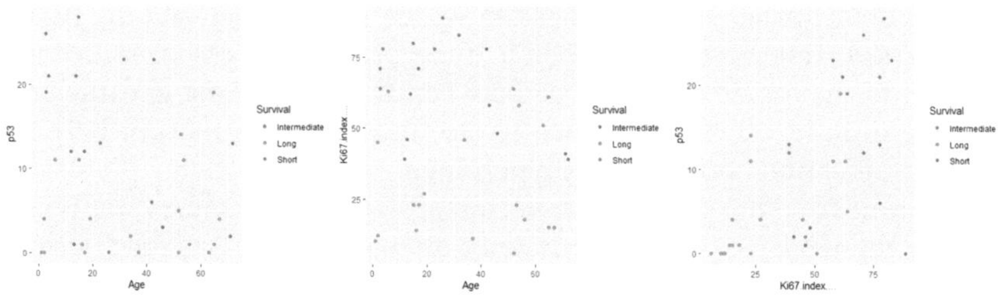

FIGURE 9.1 Scatter plot of numeric variables with respect to patients' survival.

The position of a data point in relation to the hyperplane and the margin determines its class. This is based on the binary output of the cost (loss) function. In this function, if the predicted class of a data point and the actual class are the same, the output of the function will be 0; otherwise, we need to calculate the loss for that data point:

$$c\big(x, y, f(x)\big) = \begin{cases} 0, \text{ if } y * f(x) \geq 1 \\ 1 - y * f(x), \text{else} \end{cases} \tag{9.2}$$

where y is the actual value and $f(x)$ is the predicted value that determines the class. In order to balance the loss and the maximization in the cost function, a regularization parameter is added to the cost function, making the cost function for the SVM model as

$$\min_w \lambda ||w||^2 + \sum_{i=1}^{n} \big(1 - y_i x_i, w\big). \tag{9.3}$$

The cost function is an important aspect of the SVM model, as it can control the extent to which our model can be flexible in making a prediction for unseen data. The cost function penalizes for the misclassifications and errors made by the model. Therefore, a larger cost parameter results in a better prediction of unseen data. In order to optimize this nonlinear equation, we use the Karush–Kuhn–Tucker (KKT) conditions to optimize the equation and minimize the loss. By applying the KKT condition, the weight vector is given as follows:

$$w = \sum_{i=1}^{n} \alpha_i y_i x_i \tag{9.4}$$

where similar to linear regression, α_i denotes unknown parameters for each data point. α_i can vary for each data point and determine the effect of that data point on the model and decision boundary. For some data points, α_i equals 0, meaning those data points have no effect on the final decision boundary. From Eqs. (9.1) and (9.4), we have:

$$f(x) = \text{sign}\left(\sum_{i \in \text{SV}} \alpha_i y_i K(x, x_i) + b\right) \tag{9.5}$$

where SV are the support vectors. In this equation, $K\big(x_i, x_j\big) = \phi(x_i).\phi(x_j)$, where $\phi(x)$ is called the kernel function and is defined as the dot product of features in the feature space. The parameters of the function are updated every time a data point is classified, trying to optimize the regularization parameters.

Hands-on support vector machine in R

We briefly overviewed the calculations behind SVM classifiers. In this section, we use SVM and SVR for the prediction of classes and values, respectively, using the data sets from Chapter 7.

In order to make the SVM classifier, we need to first import the data, which in this case is the data represented in Table 7.3. We call this data set "data_SVM."

```
> head(data_SVM)
  Age Stage Ki67.index.... p53     Survival
1  42     3             78   6 Intermediate
2   2     1             12   0         Long
3  34     2             46   2         Long
4   6     2             63  11         Long
5  32     2             83  23        Short
6  15     4             80  28        Short
```

Similar to the previous chapters, we need to make sure that our features are being represented by the object class we intended for them to be and make the necessary changes. In this case, we need the output variable as well as the stage of the disease to be a factor variable.

```
> str(data_SVM)
'data.frame':   36 obs. of  5 variables:
 $ Age           : int  42 2 34 6 32 15 65 23 63 13 ...
 $ Stage         : int  3 1 2 2 2 4 2 4 3 2 ...
 $ Ki67.index....: int  78 12 46 63 83 80 15 78 51 46 ...
 $ p53           : int  6 0 2 11 23 28 1 13 0 1 ...
 $ Survival      : chr  "Intermediate" "Long" "Long" "Long" ...
> data_SVM$Stage <- as.factor(data_SVM$Stage)
> data_SVM$Survival <- as.factor(data_SVM$Survival)
```

```
> str(data_SVM)
'data.frame':   36 obs. of  5 variables:
 $ Age           : int  42 2 34 6 32 15 65 23 63 13 ...
 $ Stage         : Factor w/ 4 levels "1","2","3","4": 3 1 2 2 2 4 2 4 3 2 ..
.
 $ Ki67.index....: int  78 12 46 63 83 80 15 78 51 46 ...
 $ p53           : int  6 0 2 11 23 28 1 13 0 1 ...
 $ Survival      : Factor w/ 3 levels "Intermediate",..: 1 2 2 2 3 3 2 1 2 1
...
```

We have seen the relationship between the variables by plotting pairs of variables (Fig. 7.4). Let us investigate the relationship between numeric variables with respect to the survival of patients by visualizing the scatter plots using the qplot( ) function from the "ggplot2" package [4]. We will have three pairs of variables to plot. In order to have all three variables in a single plot, we profit from the grid.arrange() function from the "gridExtra" package [5] (Fig. 9.1).

```
> install.packages("gridExtra")
> library(gridExtra)
> library(ggplot2)
> plot1<- qplot(Age, p53, data=data_SVM, color= Survival)
> plot2<- qplot(Age, Ki67.index...., data=data_SVM, color= Survival)
> plot3<- qplot(Ki67.index...., p53, data=data_SVM, color= Survival)
> grid.arrange(plot1, plot2, plot3, nrow=1)
```

By inspecting the scatter plots shown in Fig. 9.1, we can predict that the survival of patients may not be well categorized based on the numeric variables as there is no clear delineation between the dots representing the three survival categories. Having this in mind, we move forward with creating our SVM classifier. In this chapter, we make two classifiers. One is based on the entire data set, which we name SVM1, which can be used for other data sets with similar variables. The other classifier, SVM2, will be trained based on a training subset of the data set. Obviously, the model that will be trained based on the entire data set is more likely to have better accuracy; however, we can test the performance of the SVM2 model using the data set in hand, which offsets the smaller training data.

In order to make the SVM classifiers, we use the "e1071" package [6], one of the most commonly used packages for making SVM classifiers in R.

```
> install.packages("e1071")
> library(e1071)
```

Similar to what we did in the previous chapter, in order to be able to compare the performance of different algorithms on the same data set, we use all the independent variables to train our model:

```
> SVM1 <- svm(Survival~., data=data_SVM)
> summary(SVM1)

Call:
svm(formula = Survival ~ ., data = data_SVM)


Parameters:
   SVM-Type:  C-classification
 SVM-Kernel:  radial
       cost:  1

Number of Support Vectors:  26

 ( 8 11 7 )


Number of Classes:  3

Levels:
 Intermediate Long Short
```

NOTE...

We can change the kernel function used for making our classifier. There are four possibilities for the kernel argument in the svm() function of the package "e1071": "linear," "polynomial," "sigmoid," and "radial basis," which is the default function for this argument. We can try different kernel functions to evaluate their effects on the performance of our model. Later in this chapter, we will make alternatives to our SVM1 model using different kernel functions and compare the accuracy of the four models.

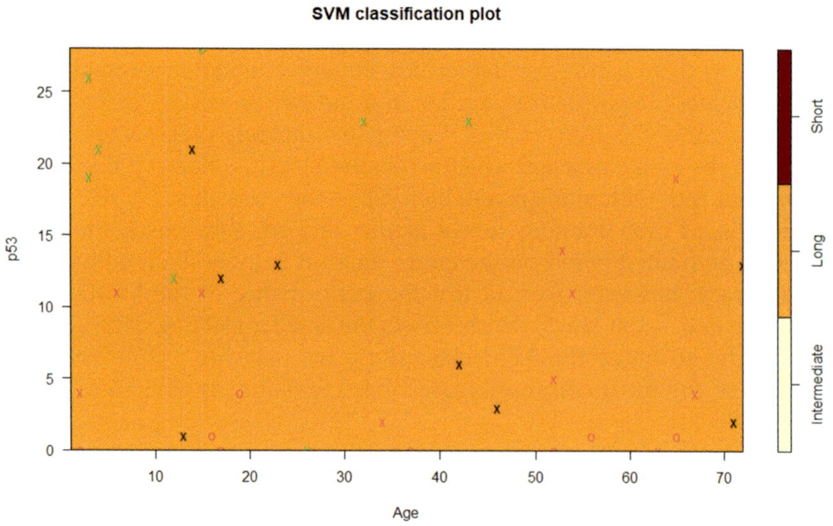

FIGURE 9.2 SVM plot of p53 against age. Support vectors are shown by X.

In the summary of the model, we are presented with some basic information regarding the model. The SVM-Type is classification as our dependent variable is a factor variable. SVM-Kernel determines which type of kernel function is used to train the model. As a default, this argument is set to "radial"; however, this can be changed to find better fits for the SVM model trained on our data set. Cost is the parameter determining the cost of constraint violation and penalizing misclassification, and by default, it is set to 1. In the summary, we also see the number of support vectors that determine our decision boundary. In our model, 8 of the support vectors are of the class "Intermediate," 11 of the class "Long," and 7 of the class "Short."

In order to have a better understanding of our model and how it can classify data points, we plot our model (Figs. 9.2–9.4).

```
> Mplot1 <- plot(SVM1, data=data_SVM,
+                p53~Age,
+                slice=list(Ki67.index....=3, Stage=3))
> Mplot2 <- plot(SVM1, data=data_SVM,
+                Ki67.index....~Age,
+                slice=list(p53=3, Stage=3))
> Mplot3 <- plot(SVM1, data=data_SVM,
+                p53~Ki67.index....,
+                slice=list(Age=3, Stage=3))
```

Even though the SVM model takes into consideration all variables irrespective of their class, plotting the model only takes two numeric variables on each plot. In order to do so, we need to set the independent variables not represented on the two axes of the plot to a constant. This constant is determined through the "slice" argument of the plot function in the "e1071"

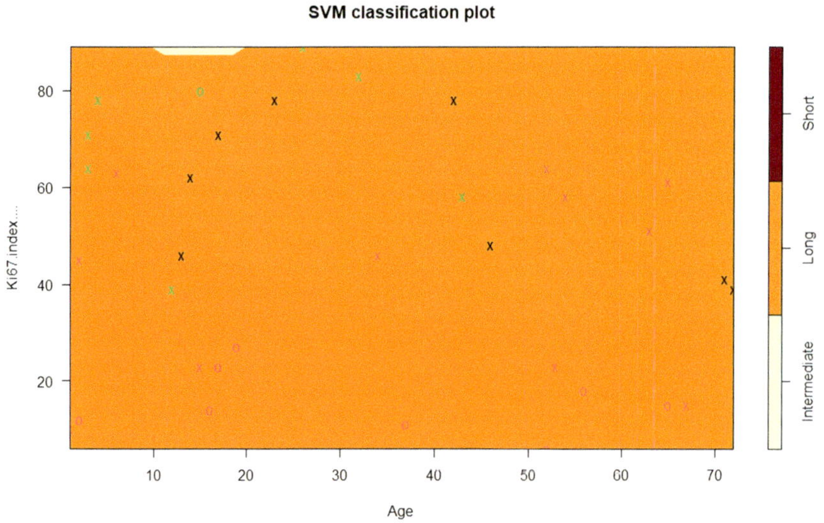

FIGURE 9.3 SVM plot of the Ki67 index against age. Support vectors are shown by X.

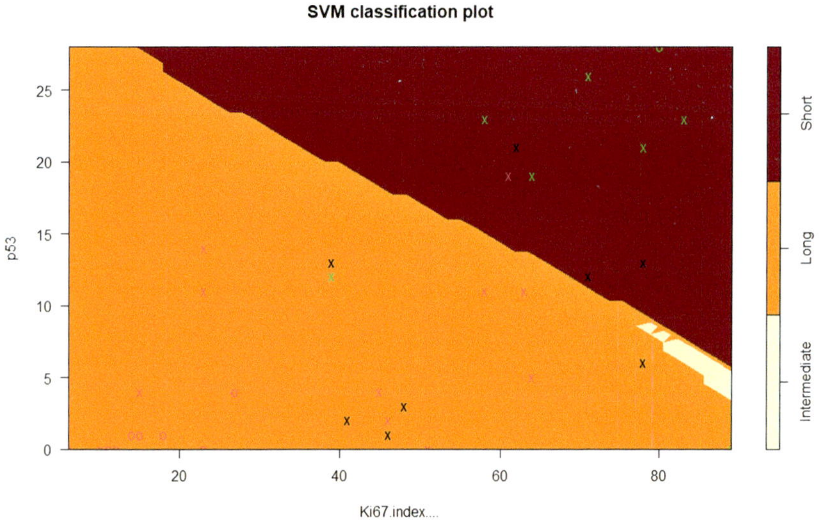

FIGURE 9.4 SVM plot of p53 against the Ki67 index. Support vectors are shown by X.

package. Although the value assigned to each of the variables not being plotted on the axes to set their effect to a constant can change the outline of the plot, the performance of the model is not affected by this constant, and it only affects the visualization of our model. As an example, in Fig. 9.5, if we set Ki67.index.... to 110, the decision boundaries will be more clear as the weight assigned to the variables is changed.

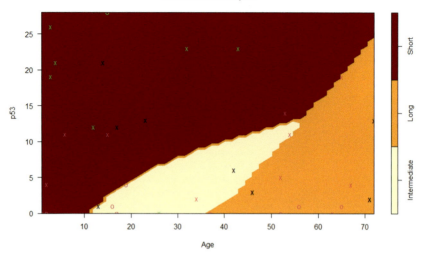

FIGURE 9.5 SVM plot of p53 against age. Support vectors are shown by X. Change of the constant values assigned to each of the features not shown in the plot (here, Ki67. index.... = 110) can alter the outline of the plot but not the performance of the model.

NOTE...

We can only plot numeric variables against one another when plotting SVM. This is due to the fact that mathematical operations, such as summing, finding the minimum or maximum value, etc., are not applicable to factor variables, and therefore, it is not possible to plot them against one another or against numeric variables in SVM.

```
> plot(SVM1, data=data_SVM,
+       p53~Stage,
+       slice=list(Ki67.index....=110, Age=1))
Error in Summary.factor(c(3L, 1L, 2L, 2L, 2L, 4L, 2L, 4L, 3L, 2L,
1L,  :
  'min' not meaningful for factors
```

As could be predicted from the scatter plot of our data, color-coded based on the patients' survival, sharp boundaries cannot be achieved to separate the classes of the outcome. The plot of our model confirms this regarding the efficacy of the model. However, in order to quantify the accuracy and performance of the model in determining the class of the dependent variable, we use the confusion matrix.

```
> prediction <- predict(SVM1, data_SVM)
> ConfusionMatrix <- table(predicted=prediction, actual=data_SVM$Survival)
> ConfusionMatrix
              actual
predicted      Intermediate Long Short
  Intermediate            3    1     0
  Long                    3   19     1
  Short                   2    0     7
```

Before calculating the accuracy of the model, a look at the confusion matrix shows a trend toward misclassifying data points as the "Long" category, which can be justified by the fact that the number of support vectors belonging to the "Long" category was higher than the two other classes. Similar to what we did in the previous chapter to calculate the accuracy from the confusion matrix, we divide the sum of numbers on the diagonal (correctly classified data points) by the sum of all the numbers in the matrix (all data points).

```
> sum(diag(ConfusionMatrix))/sum(ConfusionMatrix)
[1] 0.8055556
```

The accuracy of predictions is acceptable in terms of percentage. We can test other kernel functions to understand the effects of the kernel function on the model's accuracy. For demonstration purposes, we try to make an SVM classifier using the polynomial kernel function and compare the accuracies of the two models:

```
> svm_polynomial<-svm(Survival~., data=data_SVM, kernel="polynomial")
> summary(svm_polynomial)

Call:
svm(formula = Survival ~ ., data = data_SVM, kernel = "polynomial")


Parameters:
   SVM-Type:  C-classification
 SVM-Kernel:  polynomial
       cost:  1
     degree:  3
     coef.0:  0

Number of Support Vectors:  26

 ( 8 11 7 )


Number of Classes:  3

Levels:
 Intermediate Long Short
```

By taking a look at the documentation of the svm() function, we see that the two parameters added to the summary of the model, "degree" and "coef.0," are parameters used in the polynomial SVM algorithms, which are by default set to 3 and 0, respectively.

```
> prediction <- predict(svm_polynomial, data_SVM)
> ConfusionMatrix <- table(predicted=prediction, actual=data_SVM$Survival)
> ConfusionMatrix
              actual
predicted      Intermediate Long Short
  Intermediate            0    0     0
  Long                    8   20     4
  Short                   0    0     4
> sum(diag(ConfusionMatrix))/sum(ConfusionMatrix)
[1] 0.6666667
```

Taking a look at the results, we decipher that the SVM1 model made using the radial kernel function had better performance. However, taking a closer look at the confusion matrix, we observe a notable tendency to misclassify the "Intermediate" class as "Long" survival. Such selective misclassification must be considered when deciding about the performance of the models. In this case, even if the accuracy of the polynomial model was better in terms of percentage, it would still not be considered a good model for future use.

We now move on to making our second classification model by dividing the data set into training and testing subsets:

```
> set.seed(123)
> subsets <- sample(2, nrow(data_SVM), prob=c(0.7, 0.3), replace=T)
> train_SVM <- data_SVM[subsets==1,]
> test_SVM <- data_SVM[subsets==2,]
> dim(train_SVM)
[1] 23  5
```

Now, we train the model based on the training subset, consisting of 23 observations.

```
> SVM2 <- svm(Survival~., data=train_SVM)
> summary(SVM2)

Call:
svm(formula = Survival ~ ., data = train_SVM)


Parameters:
   SVM-Type:  C-classification
 SVM-Kernel:  radial
       cost:  1

Number of Support Vectors:  17

 ( 5 7 5 )


Number of Classes:  3

Levels:
 Intermediate Long Short
```

Of the 23 data points in the training subset, 17 affected the decision boundary. In order to understand the efficacy of our model, we predict the class of the dependent variable in the test subset.

```
> test_prediction <- predict(SVM2, test_SVM)
> ConfusionMatrix_test <- table(Predicted=test_prediction, Actual=test_SVM$Su
rvival)
> ConfusionMatrix_test
              Actual
Predicted      Intermediate Long Short
  Intermediate            0    1     0
  Long                    1    7     0
  Short                   2    0     2
> sum(diag(ConfusionMatrix_test))/sum(ConfusionMatrix_test)
[1] 0.6923077
```

Considering the size of the training and test data sets, making a decision regarding the accuracy of the model and misclassification biases is hard. However, as we expected, the performance of the model in predicting the class of the patients' survival is not as good as that of the SVM1. In addition to increasing the size of the training sample, altering the kernel function used, or feature selection, there are other ways of improving the performance of an SVM model, which we will learn about in Chapter 14.

Support vector regression

As mentioned earlier, the support vector can be used for both classification and regression problems. Thus far, we have learned only one regression algorithm, that is, linear regression. Linear regression attempts to find the line best fitting all data points and does so by minimizing the residual sum of squares. Therefore, it takes into account all data points. However, SVR, similar to the SVM classifier, does not take into account all data points but support vectors. SVR allows for a margin of error, data points that are close to these margins are considered support vectors, and their distance from the margin determines model predictions. Similar to the SVM classifier, these support vectors try to minimize the cost function. There are certain advantages to SVR over linear regression. SVR, being a nonparametric algorithm, does not consider the many assumptions of simple linear regression. Therefore, its performance can be better than linear regression in cases where the data set does not fulfill the assumptions of the linear regression. However, it must be noted that these features do not necessarily lead to better performance of SVR over linear regression in all cases [7].

In order to compare the performance of SVR and linear regression, we use the data set presented in Table 7.1. We had investigated the conformity of the structure of the data set with the assumptions of linear regression in Chapter 7, and we know that our data set conforms to most of the linear regression assumptions. For comparison reasons, we recreate the linear regression from Chapter 7 and a new SVR model.

We need to first import the data set and take a look at its structure to make the necessary changes:

```
> head(data)
  Age Stage Ki67.index.... p53 Survival
1  42     3             78   6       13
2   2     1             12   0      102
3  34     2             46   2       43
4   6     2             63  11       12
5  32     2             83  23        5
6  15     4             80  28        1
> str(data)
'data.frame':   36 obs. of  5 variables:
 $ Age           : int  42 2 34 6 32 15 65 23 63 13 ...
 $ Stage         : int  3 1 2 2 2 4 2 4 3 2 ...
 $ Ki67.index....: int  78 12 46 63 83 80 15 78 51 46 ...
 $ p53           : int  6 0 2 11 23 28 1 13 0 1 ...
 $ Survival      : int  13 102 43 12 5 1 45 7 41 23 ...
```

We can see that Stage is being considered as an integer, which is not what is expected. Therefore, we need to change this variable to a factor variable:

```
> data$Stage <- as.factor(data$Stage)
```

We had investigated the relationship between the variables of this data set in Fig. 7.4. Therefore, we jump straight to making the models. We need to first divide our data set into training and test subsets:

```
> set.seed(123)
> subsets <- sample(2, nrow(data), prob=c(0.7, 0.3), replace=T)
> train <- data[subsets==1,]
> test <- data[subsets==2,]
```

We start by recalling the linear regression model. We train the data using the training subset and test its performance using the test subset:

```
> linear <- lm(Survival~., data=train)
> predict_lm <- predict(linear, test)
```

We recall that in order to compare the performance of different regression models, we use root mean square error (RMSE). In Chapter 7, we learned how to calculate the RMSE; now, we use the rmse() function from the "Metrics" package to calculate the RMSE for our models:

```
> install.packages("Metrics")
> library(Metrics)
> RMSE_lm <- rmse(predict_lm, test$Survival)
> RMSE_lm
[1] 12.46179
```

We now move on to creating the SVR model. Again, we use the svm() function from the "e1071" package. The structure of the data set automatically changes the SVM-Type from classification to regression:

```
> SVR <- svm(Survival~., data=train)
> summary(SVR)

Call:
svm(formula = Survival ~ ., data = train)


Parameters:
   SVM-Type:  eps-regression
 SVM-Kernel:  radial
       cost:  1
      gamma:  0.2
    epsilon:  0.1


Number of Support Vectors:  22
```

In this summary, as no arguments of the function were altered, the epsilon value, which is a parameter in the loss function, is set as default. Gamma depends on the dimensions of the data set the model is trained upon and is calculated as 1 divided by the dimension of the data set. A look at the summary of the model shows that of the 23 data points in the training subset, 22 were used to train the model. Even though this is a considerable proportion of the training data, the linear regression used more data points to find the best fit. We need to assess the performance of the SVR model:

```
> predict_SVR <- predict(SVR, test)
> RMSE_SVR <- rmse(predict_SVR, test$Survival)
> RMSE_SVR
[1] 21.74019
```

A comparison of the RMSE of the two models shows that the performance of the simple linear regression in this data set is better than that of the SVR. Even though SVR is one of the most robust and useful regression models and has several advantages over linear regression, we must bear in mind the strength points of linear regression. Despite certain parameters in the SVR to avoid overfitting, including the loss function, the simplicity of the linear regression can perform a better job of avoiding the overfitting of the model. A more complex structure of an algorithm can result in some level of overfitting by nature, compared to simpler models. Therefore, simpler models can perform better at predicting unseen data, which can be the case here. Another factor that contributes to better performance of the linear regression is the fact that our data fulfills the assumptions of the linear regression model, which, given the robustness of the linear regression because of its simplicity, leads to better performance of the linear regression over the SVR.

References

[1] S. Huang, N. Cai, P.P. Pacheco, S. Narrandes, Y. Wang, W. Xu, Applications of support vector machine (SVM) learning in cancer genomics, Cancer Genomics & Proteomics 15 (1) (2018) 41−51.

[2] N.B. Larson, J. Chen, D.J. Schaid, A review of kernel methods for genetic association studies, Genetic Epidemiology 43 (2) (2019) 122−136.

[3] Y. Shihong, L. Ping, H. Peiyi, SVM classification: its contents and challenges, Applied Mathematics—A Journal of Chinese Universities 18 (2003) 332−342.

[4] H. Wickham, ggplot2: Elegant Graphics for Data Analysis, Springer-Verlag, New York, 2016ISBN 978-3-319-24277-4. Available from: https://ggplot2.tidyverse.org.

[5] B. Auguie, A. Antonov, gridExtra: Miscellaneous Functions for "Grid" Graphics, 2017.

[6] D. Meyer, E. Dimitriadou, K. Hornik, A. Weingessel, F. Leisch, C.C. Chang, et al., e1071: Misc Functions of the Department of Statistics, Probability Theory Group (Formerly: E1071), TU Wien, 2021.

[7] S. Kavitha, S. Varuna, R. Ramya, A comparative analysis on linear regression and support vector regression. Computer Science, 2016.

CHAPTER

10

Decision trees in R

Introduction to decision trees

Decision trees are one of the supervised learning algorithms used for both regression and classification problems. There are different algorithms that can be used to create decision tree models: iterative dichotomiser 3 (ID3), C4.5, C5.0, and classification and regression tree (CART), chi-square automatic interaction detection (CHAID), and multivariate adaptive regression splines (MARS) [1]. Similar to other supervised learning algorithms, these algorithms try to predict the class or the numerical value of the dependent variable based on the observed patterns in their input data. One of the strength points of such algorithms is that they do not restrict the variables to be numerical or categorical. In this chapter, we will discuss the more common algorithm to train decision trees, ID3.

We have seen examples of decision trees in several daily instances, specifically for classification purposes. Basically, any flowchart we have encountered is a decision tree algorithm trying to classify events. A key feature of these flowcharts is that they are supposed to be as simple as possible, meaning classifying events with the least condition settings as possible [1]. In order to realize this goal, we try to use features, and basically ask questions, that yield in better placement of events to groups in a way that events categorized into a specific group are as homogeneous as possible. As an example, consider trying to classify lymphocytes into B cells and T cells. We know that T cells are not only $CD3^+$ (cluster of differentiation 3) but can also have CD4 and CD8 along with other CD markers on their surface. On the other hand, B cells have CD19, along with CD20 and CD21, etc., on their surface. As there is no overlap between the named B and T cell markers, we can use any of these markers to classify cells as B or T cells. However, if we

DOI: https://doi.org/10.1016/B978-0-12-822400-7.00007-5

try to classify T cells into different subsets, which of the CD markers would be helpful given that CD3 is common among helper and cytotoxic T cells? It is clear that using CD3 to classify T cells will not yield in a good classification, as we will end up with our starting samples. This concept is reflected in "information gain" in decision tree algorithms which will be explained in detail when overviewing the mathematics behind decision trees [2].

Before we move on to how decision tree algorithms work and practice with the hands-on examples in R, let us review the terminology behind decision trees. Each decision tree has a root node (Fig. 10.1) that encompasses the entire data set. This root node is then divided into two or more sub-nodes through the splitting process. The splitting process is basically the question asked (here, the feature considered) that can split the data into two or more homogeneous groups in a way that we have the highest level of information gain. If a sub-node can be further divided into more sub-nodes, it is called a "decision node"; however, if it cannot be further divided, the sub-node is a terminal node. Ideally, terminal nodes are homogenous; however, depending on the level of information gain with further branching, terminal nodes can include more than one class of data [1].

We mentioned earlier that what determines which of the features should be used for splitting of nodes is homogeneity of samples in each of

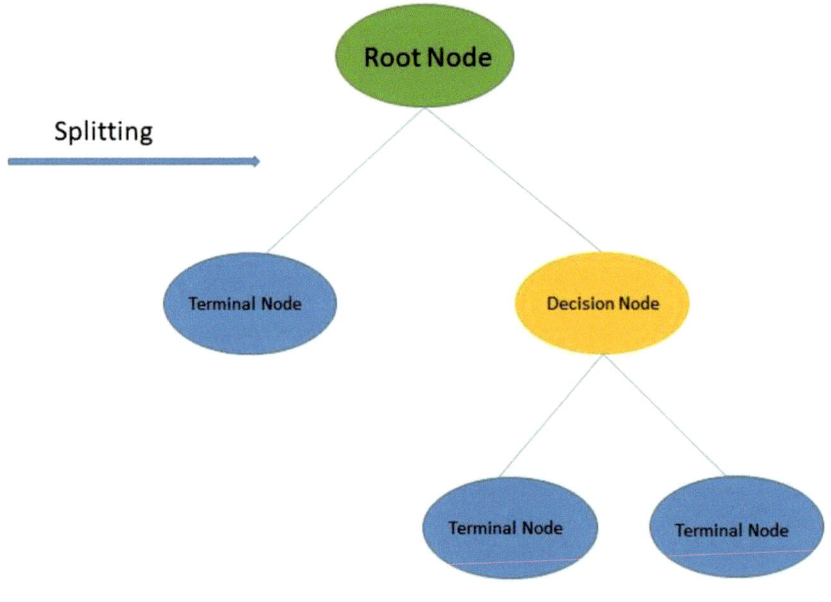

FIGURE 10.1 A simple decision tree and the associated terminology.

the resulting sub-nodes and information gain. Information gain has a negative correlation with entropy after transforming a data set. In other words, information gain is the reduction in entropy after we divide the data set based on a variable. Entropy determines the level of heterogeneity in a group. If all samples assigned to a group are the same or very similar, entropy in that group is zero or close to zero. On the other hand, if the sample is equally divided into two different groups, the entropy equals 1, which is the highest value for entropy in a dichotomous situation [1] (Fig. 10.2). However, in multiclass data sets, entropy can be greater than 1, and the more heterogeneous a sample is, the higher the entropy value will be (10.1). Entropy for a sample with "c" classes is calculated as:

$$E = \sum_{i=1}^{c} - p_i \log_2^{p_i}, \tag{10.1}$$

where p_i is the probability of class i. However, this only accounts for the probabilities of two events in the sample. As an example, what is the entropy for a group including 100 T cells and 120 B cells. If we aim to divide the instances based on an attribute, like CD markers, we need to calculate the entropy with the following equation:

$$E(A, B) = \sum_{c=B} P(c)E(c) \tag{10.2}$$

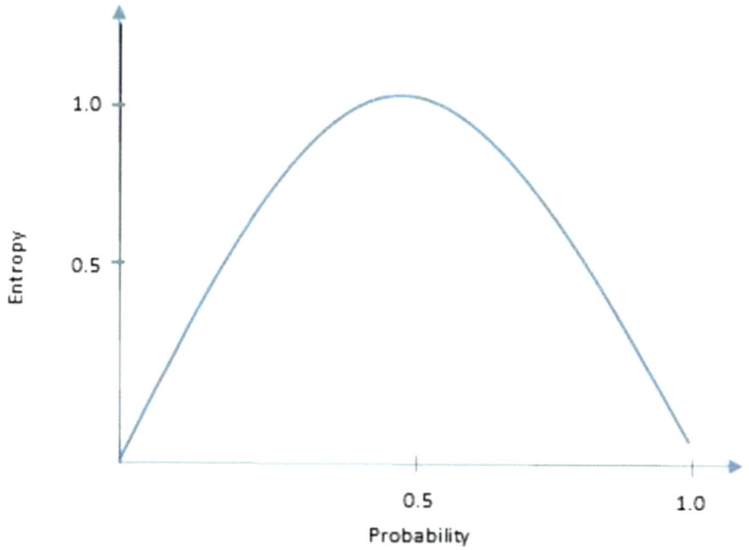

FIGURE 10.2 The association between entropy and probability in a binary classification. Equal probabilities for the two classes result in the highest entropy.

As an example, entropy for $CD4^+$ T cells based on the following table of attributes would be calculated as follows:

		Lymphocytes		
		T cells	B cells	
CD marker	CD4	30	0	30
	CD8	70	0	70
	CD19	0	80	80
	CD20	0	40	40
		100	120	220

$$E(T\,cell, CD\,marker) = \sum_{c\,=\,CD\,marker} P(c)E(c)$$

$$= P(CD4)E(30, 0) + P(CD8)E(70, 0) + P(CD19)E(0, 80) + P(CD20)E(0, 40)$$

This helps us find the entropy for CD marker attribute. In a data set with more attributes, we calculate the entropy for each of the attributes following the example above, and the attribute with the highest information gain based on the following equation is used to split the node into further sub-nodes, until all samples are divided into homogeneous sub-nodes, if possible:

$$Gain(A, B) = E(A) - E(A, B) \tag{10.3}$$

Hands-on decision trees in R

As mentioned earlier, decision trees can be used for both classification and regression problems. In this chapter, we use the data set that was used in previous chapters for creating classification and regression models, as also presented in Tables 7.1 and 7.3.

We start off by creating the decision tree classifier. Similar to previous chapters, we first import the data and check the structure of our data set to make sure that variable classes match our purposes for classification:

```
> str(data)
'data.frame':   36 obs. of  5 variables:
 $ Age         : int  42 2 34 6 32 15 65 23 63 13 ...
 $ Stage       : int  3 1 2 2 2 4 2 4 3 2 ...
 $ Ki67.index....: int  78 12 46 63 83 80 15 78 51 46 ...
 $ p53         : int  6 0 2 11 23 28 1 13 0 1 ...
 $ Survival    : chr  "Intermediate" "Long" "Long" "Long" ...
```

Age, Ki67 index, and p53 are recognized as integers, which given their numeric nature are consistent with their expected class. However, patients' survival groups and their disease stages are recognized as character and integers which are not consistent with our background knowledge of their role in our analyses. Therefore, we need to change these variables to factor variables:

```
> data$Survival <- as.factor(data$Survival)
> data$Stage <- as.factor(data$Stage)
> str(data)
'data.frame':   36 obs. of  5 variables:
 $ Age            : int  42 2 34 6 32 15 65 23 63 13 ...
 $ Stage          : Factor w/ 4 levels "1","2","3","4": 3 1 2 2 2 4 2 4 3 2 ..
.
 $ Ki67.index....: int  78 12 46 63 83 80 15 78 51 46 ...
 $ p53            : int  6 0 2 11 23 28 1 13 0 1 ...
 $ Survival       : Factor w/ 3 levels "Intermediate",..: 1 2 2 2 3 3 2 1 2 1
...
```

We can now split our data set to training and testing subsets. For this purpose, similar to previous chapters, we use 70% of our data for training and spare 30% for testing the accuracy of our model. Also, bear in mind that since we want to compare the accuracy of the decision tree algorithm with that of the classifiers from previous chapters, we need to keep all the parameters in division of the data set to training and test subsets as previous chapters:

```
> set.seed(123)
> subsets <- sample(2, nrow(data), prob=c(0.7, 0.3), replace=T)
> train <- data[subsets==1,]
> test <- data[subsets==2,]
```

We now have the material needed to create our classifier tree. Even though there are several packages that can be used to create decision trees, we choose to create our classifier tree using one of the simplest packages dedicated to creating decision trees, the "party" package [3]:

```
> install.packages("party")
> library(party)
```

This package can be used for creating the Random Forest algorithm in addition to the Decision Tree algorithm. In order to create the classifier tree, we use the ctree() function (10.3). We call our decision tree model DT, and similar to what we did with the logistic regression model, we use all the variables for training our model:

```
> DT <- ctree(data$Survival~., data=train)
> DT

         Conditional inference tree with 2 terminal nodes

Response:  Survival
Inputs:  Age, Stage, Ki67.index...., p53
Number of observations:  23

1) Ki67.index.... <= 23; criterion = 0.991, statistic = 14.911
  2)*  weights = 8
1) Ki67.index.... > 23
  3)*  weights = 15
```

Based on the information on our decision tree, we can see that there are overall three nodes in our model. Also, we can see that only Ki67 index is used for classification here as it has the highest correlation with the group of data points. In order to interpret our plot easily, we create our decision tree (Fig. 10.3; Table 10.1).

```
> plot(DT)
```

The terminal nodes in any decision tree, as shown in Fig. 10.3, show the probability of each class when the splitting feature is true. From this tree we understand that there were no instances of short or intermediate survival in patients whose Ki67 index was below 27. On the other hand, patients whose Ki67 index is above 27 have equal probability of belonging to either of the groups. However, this node is no further split. One of the possible reasons is that there is no information gain if further splitting occurs, or that the information gain would be equal for all the possible features.

We can have an estimate of how good our decision tree might perform in classifying data points by looking at its structure. Our decision tree classifier used only one variable for determining the class of data. On the other hand, one of the terminal nodes is not homogeneous. These suggest a simple, however, less accurate model. In order to compare the performance of our decision tree classifier with other classifiers, we need to find out its exact accuracy in classifying unseen data,

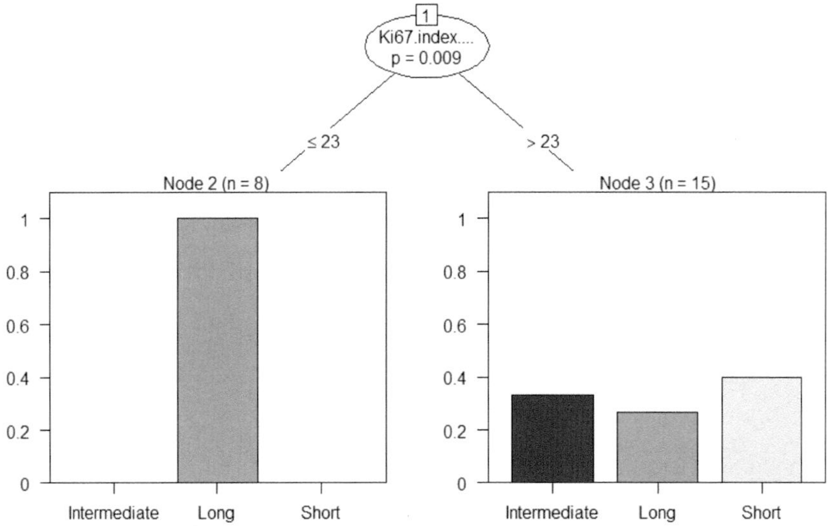

FIGURE 10.3 Decision tree trained by a subset of the data presented in Table 10.1 using the ID3 algorithm.

here the testing subset. For this purpose, similar to previous chapters, we use the confusion matrix. Remember that we still need to evaluate the accuracy of our model in the face of new data, here the testing subset. For this purpose, we use the predict() function which can also show the probability of each data point belonging to one of the classes using this function:

```
> predict_prob <- predict(DT, test, type="prob")
> predict_prob
[[1]]
[1] 0 1 0

[[2]]
[1] 0.3333333 0.2666667 0.4000000

[[3]]
[1] 0.3333333 0.2666667 0.4000000

[[4]]
[1] 0.3333333 0.2666667 0.4000000

[[5]]
[1] 0.3333333 0.2666667 0.4000000

[[6]]
[1] 0 1 0

[[7]]
[1] 0.3333333 0.2666667 0.4000000

[[8]]
[1] 0.3333333 0.2666667 0.4000000

[[9]]
[1] 0 1 0

[[10]]
[1] 0 1 0

[[11]]
[1] 0.3333333 0.2666667 0.4000000

[[12]]
[1] 0.3333333 0.2666667 0.4000000


[[13]]
[1] 0.3333333 0.2666667 0.4000000
> predict <- predict(DT, test)
> predict
 [1] Long  Short Short Short Short Long  Short Short Long  Long  Short Short
Short
Levels: Intermediate Long Short
> ConfusionMatrix=table(test$Survival,predict)
> ConfusionMatrix
              predict
               Intermediate Long Short
  Intermediate            0    0     3
  Long                    0    4     4
  Short                   0    0     2
> sum(diag(ConfusionMatrix))/sum(ConfusionMatrix)
[1] 0.4615385
```

As was predicted, the accuracy of the model is not as high as previous classifiers for the reasons mentioned earlier. While with other classification models we had more freedom in deciding what independent variables to include in the model, decision trees automatically omit some of the variables from the classification algorithm. Even though

TABLE 10.1 Imaginary data on the survival of neuroblastoma patients.

Age	Stage	Ki67 index (%)	p53	Survival
42	3	78	6	Intermediate
2	1	12	0	Long
34	2	46	2	Long
6	2	63	11	Long
32	2	83	23	Short
15	4	80	28	Short
65	2	15	1	Long
23	4	78	13	Intermediate
63	3	51	0	Long
13	2	46	1	Intermediate
19	1	27	4	Long
54	2	58	11	Long
72	4	39	13	Intermediate
3	3	71	26	Short
14	3	62	21	Intermediate
56	2	18	1	Long
2	1	45	4	Long
43	4	58	23	Short
16	2	14	1	Long
17	3	71	12	Intermediate
52	2	64	5	Long
17	2	23	0	Long
26	2	89	0	Short
53	1	23	14	Long
1	1	10	0	Long
52	1	6	0	Long
71	3	41	2	Intermediate
4	4	78	21	Short
15	2	23	11	Long
67	1	15	4	Long

(Continued)

TABLE 10.1 (Continued)

Age	Stage	Ki67 index (%)	p53	Survival
3	3	64	19	Short
46	3	48	3	Intermediate
17	2	23	0	Long
65	4	61	19	Long
37	1	11	0	Long
12	3	39	12	Short

this omission of variables can have detrimental effects on smaller data sets, they can be useful for data sets with large dimensions. Higher number of variables can usually favor our model; however, it can sometimes be at the expense of model complexity and speed of performing calculations for larger data sets. Therefore, in the instance of larger data sets with several variables, the use of decision tree algorithms can yield better accuracy as these are stricter with the inclusion of variables to train the models.

Decision trees for regression

Decision tree regression is very similar to decision tree classifiers. In the regression algorithm, the decision on branching a node is made by using reduction in standard deviation for each node, instead of information gain. Decision tree regression, similar to support vector regression, allows for nonlinearity of the correlations between the attributes and the target variable [4]. Therefore, it can be useful for data sets that do not conform to the assumption of the simple linear regression model. However, as we noticed in Chapter 7, the increased level of complexity for these models compared to that of simple linear regression can lead to poorer performance in predicting unseen continuous variables. Even though decision trees are among the common regression algorithms with acceptable robustness for any data set, their use is best reserved for categorical independent features. In instances where the independent features are continuous, and the data do not conform to assumptions of linear regression, support vector regression may perform a better job of making predictions.

In order to compare the performance of decision trees in predicting continuous variables, with that of the linear regression and support vector regression, we use the data set presented in Table 7.1. Similar to previous chapters, we need to make sure the structure of the data set is as required:

```
> str(reg_data)
'data.frame':   36 obs. of  5 variables:
 $ Age           : int  42 2 34 6 32 15 65 23 63 13 ...
 $ Stage         : int  3 1 2 2 2 4 2 4 3 2 ...
 $ Ki67.index....: int  78 12 46 63 83 80 15 78 51 46 ...
 $ p53           : int  6 0 2 11 23 28 1 13 0 1 ...
 $ Survival      : int  13 102 43 12 5 1 45 7 41 23 ...
> reg_data$Stage <- as.factor(reg_data$Stage)
```

Now we divide our data set into the training and testing subsets using the same parameters used in the previous chapters:

```
> set.seed(123)
> subsets <- sample(2, nrow(reg_data), prob=c(0.7, 0.3), replace=T)
> reg_train <- reg_data[subsets==1,]
> reg_test <- reg_data[subsets==2,]
```

Even though the same package used for creating decision tree classifier can be used to make decision tree regression models, we will use a simpler package, called "tree," [5] for making the latter.

```
> install.packages("tree")
> library(tree)
```

Now we train our model, which we will name "reg_DT" using the training subset:

```
> reg_DT <- tree(Survival~., data=reg_train)
> reg_DT
node), split, n, deviance, yval
      * denotes terminal node

1) root 23 16270.0 32.350
  2) Ki67.index.... < 31 8  4345.0 59.880 *
  3) Ki67.index.... > 31 15  2625.0 17.670
    6) p53 < 11.5 8  1310.0 26.000 *
    7) p53 > 11.5 7   124.9  8.143 *
> summary(reg_DT)
Regression tree:
tree(formula = Survival ~ ., data = reg_train)
Variables actually used in tree construction:
[1] "Ki67.index...." "p53"
Number of terminal nodes:  3
Residual mean deviance:  289 = 5780 / 20
Distribution of residuals:
   Min. 1st Qu.  Median    Mean 3rd Qu.    Max.
-32.880 -10.070  -2.143   0.000   6.500  34.120
```

A look at the summary and characteristics of the model shows us that there are a total of three terminal nodes by using "Ki67.index…." and "p53." The model has determined the cutoff values for each of these features that will be used for the branching of the nodes. A further look at each of the nodes shows more information regarding the data points placed in that node and further splitting happening at that node. As an example, we look at the third node. The following values are shown for the third node: >31, 15, 2625.0, and 17.670. The first line in the output of the results helps us interpret these numbers. The first value (here 31) shows the cutoff value for splitting. The second number, 15, is represented as "n" in the output guide, representing the number of data points in that node. Note that in nodes 2 and 3, we have all 23 data points, as they are the result of splitting from the root node. The third number, 2625.0, shows the deviance at that node. The last number, 17.670, shows the value that would be predicted for that node if there were no further splitting.

Residual mean of deviance, a representative of how good the model can make predictions, is the total residual deviance divided by the degree of freedom. The smaller the residual mean deviance of our model, the better is the performance of the model in making predictions. Other factors can also affect the number of residual deviance, including the number of variables included in the model. However, root mean square error (RMSE) remains the best parameter to compare the performance of different regression models, so we need to calculate RMSE of our reg_DT model to compare its performance to other regression models created thus far in this book. However, before comparing our models' performances, let us plot our decision tree regression model (Fig. 10.4), which can be helpful in both understanding the model and interpreting the results:

```
> plot(reg_DT)
> text(reg_DT)
```

As can be seen, there are two steps in plotting the decision tree. The first step only shows the splitting branches, and the second step adds the text to the nodes.

We now compare the performance of our model with other regression models by calculating its RMSE:

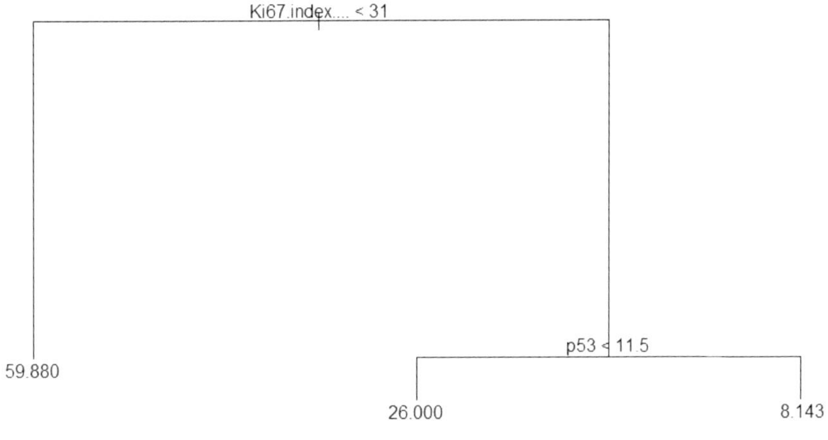

FIGURE 10.4 The plot of the decision tree regression model.

```
> predict_DT <- predict(reg_DT, test)
> RMSE_DT <- rmse(predict_DT, reg_test$Survival)
> RMSE_DT
[1] 15.7766
```

The RMSE of our model shows accuracy similar to that of the support vector regression; however, the performance is still poorer than that of the linear regression model for the same reasons as discussed in Chapter 9 [6].

The decision tree models developed in this chapter were relatively simple in terms of the number of nodes and splitting. In Chapter 14, we will encounter more complicated trees and learn how to control the complexity of the tree by changing the arguments of our functions, a process called pruning of the tree.

References

[1] C. Kingsford, S.L. Salzberg, What are decision trees? Nature Biotechnology 26 (9) (2008) 1011–1013.
[2] Y.Y. Song, Y. Lu, Decision tree methods: applications for classification and prediction, Shanghai Archives of Psychiatry 27 (2) (2015) 130–135.
[3] T. Hothorn, K. Hornik, A. Zeileis, Unbiased recursive partitioning: a conditional inference framework, Journal of Computational and Graphical Statistics 15 (3) (2006) 651–674.
[4] S.C. Lemon, J. Roy, M.A. Clark, P.D. Friedmann, W. Rakowski, Classification and regression tree analysis in public health: methodological review and comparison with logistic regression, Annals of Behavioral Medicine: A Publication of the Society of Behavioral Medicine 26 (3) (2003) 172–181.
[5] B. Ripley, Tree: Classification and Regression Trees, 2021.
[6] R. Pajouheshnia, W.R. Pestman, S. Teerenstra, R.H.H. Groenwold, A computational approach to compare regression modelling strategies in prediction research, BMC Medical Research Methodology 16 (2016) 107.

CHAPTER

11

Random forests in R

What is a random forest?

Random forest is another supervised learning algorithm that is commonly used for both regression (random forest regressors) and classification problems (random forest classifiers). As the name may suggest, random forests rely on several decision tree algorithms, hence the name forest [1]. Random forests can be considered as a committee among different decision trees concerned with a specific prediction, and the prediction made by the majority of trees in the forest determines the outcome [1].

In order to create different decision trees based on a data set, random forests use bootstrap aggregating or bagging [2]. In bagging, random subsets of our data set are selected and a decision tree is trained using each of the subsets. This results in various trees with various predictions through cross validation. The final result is the consensus of the results achieved by all trees through a majority voting system [1], a technic also known as ensemble learning. It can be deduced that an increased number of trees will result in increased accuracy of the random forest predictions. However, as will be shown later in this chapter, the increase in the number of trees will not constantly increase the accuracy model of our (Fig. 11.1).

Certain criteria must be met for random forests to perform their best. A key feature is that decision trees making a random forest are relatively uncorrelated [2]. As mentioned, the outcome agreed upon by most decision trees will be chosen as the final outcome of the random forest. Therefore, if decision trees are correlated, the results will be biased and less accurate.

DOI: https://doi.org/10.1016/B978-0-12-822400-7.00001-4

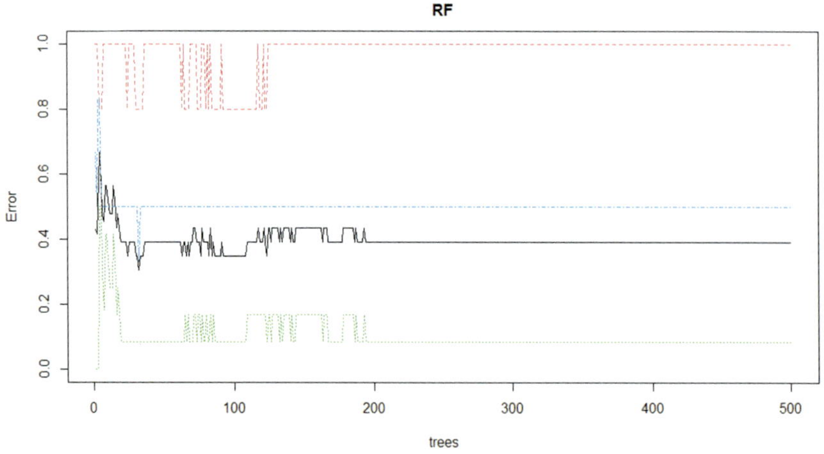

FIGURE 11.1 Random forest plot. The error rates decrease as the number of trees increases. The optimum number of trees can be determined when the error rate does not change with increase in number of trees.

Random forests have certain advantages over other predictive algorithms, especially when compared to decision trees. They can handle a large number of variables without overfitting the model [3]. Similar to decision trees, random forest algorithms can be used to find which features in our data set are more important in predicting the outcome, so they can help with feature selection for other algorithms as well [4]. We can control the efficacy of random forests to some extent by controlling different parameters of the model. Furthermore, random forests do not have several assumptions that can limit their use or their accuracy in working with real-world data. Another strength point of random forests is that they use bagging or bootstrapping to make each decision tree. This method of cross-validation allows for using all data set to train the model and result in higher accuracy.

Hands-on random forest in R

Random forest classifiers

As mentioned, the performance of a random forest is generally better than decision trees on the same data set. In order to better understand this point, we compare the performance of the random forest classifier with that of the decision tree classifier from Chapter 10 using the same data set.

Even though to train random forests we do not need to divide the data set into training and testing subsets as data are randomly bagged to train the model, in order to use the same data points as previous chapters we divide the data set into training and testing subsets to make comparison of models' performance easier. Therefore, we keep the basic parameters of creating the model the same and use 70% of the data for training the model and 30% to test the accuracy of the model facing new data. However, we remember from the previous chapters that we must check the structure of our data set before dividing it into testing and training subsets to make sure that each variable is being treated as it should be

```
> head(data)
  Age Stage Ki67.index.... p53     Survival
1  42     3             78   6 Intermediate
2   2     1             12   0         Long
3  34     2             46   2         Long
4   6     2             63  11         Long
5  32     2             83  23        Short
6  15     4             80  28        Short
```

```
> str(data)
'data.frame':   36 obs. of  5 variables:
 $ Age           : int  42 2 34 6 32 15 65 23 63 13 ...
 $ Stage         : int  3 1 2 2 2 4 2 4 3 2 ...
 $ Ki67.index....: int  78 12 46 63 83 80 15 78 51 46 ...
 $ p53           : int  6 0 2 11 23 28 1 13 0 1 ...
 $ Survival      : chr  "Intermediate" "Long" "Long" "Long" ...
```

Therefore we make sure that the "Stage" and "Survival" variables are converted to the appropriate class

```
> data$Survival <- as.factor(data$Survival)
> data$Stage <- as.factor(data$Stage)

> str(data)
'data.frame':   36 obs. of  5 variables:
 $ Age           : int  42 2 34 6 32 15 65 23 63 13 ...
 $ Stage         : Factor w/ 4 levels "1","2","3","4": 3 1 2 2 2 4 2 4 3 2 ..
.
 $ Ki67.index....: int  78 12 46 63 83 80 15 78 51 46 ...
 $ p53           : int  6 0 2 11 23 28 1 13 0 1 ...
 $ Survival      : Factor w/ 3 levels "Intermediate",..: 1 2 2 2 3 3 2 1 2 1
...
```

Then, we divide the data set into training and testing subsets

```
> set.seed(123)
> subsets <- sample(2, nrow(data), prob=c(0.7, 0.3), replace=T)
> train <- data[subsets==1,]
> test <- data[subsets==2,]
```

The previous steps were mutual between all algorithms we have seen. Now, our data are ready to be used for training a random forest model. For this purpose, we use the "randomForest" package [5]

```
> install.packages("randomForest")
> library(randomForest)
```

In this package, the default number of trees is set to 500, which can be altered by changing the "ntree" parameter. Furthermore, for each decision tree created as part of the random forest, a certain number of features are randomly chosen (m_{try}). This number is determined by the number of entire features in the data set. For random forest classifiers, this number roughly equals the square root of the number of features.

In order to get the same results when repeating the steps below, we fix the effect of randomizations using set.seed() function.

```
> set.seed(123)
> RF <- randomForest(Survival~., data=train)
> RF

Call:
 randomForest(formula = Survival ~ ., data = train)
               Type of random forest: classification
                     Number of trees: 500
No. of variables tried at each split: 2

        OOB estimate of  error rate: 39.13%
Confusion matrix:
             Intermediate Long Short class.error
Intermediate            0    2     3  1.00000000
Long                    1   11     0  0.08333333
Short                   2    1     3  0.50000000
```

As was mentioned earlier, 500 trees are created in the random forest. The number of variables tried at each split, also known as the m_{try}, is the closest integer to the square root of the four independent variables in the data set. Out-of-bag (OOB) estimate of error is how well the decision trees can predict the data points not included in their training data (bagged data). Therefore the lower the error rate, the better the predictions of our model. Even though the OOB error rate is quite high in this random forest model, this high error rate can be justified by the small size of our data set. Furthermore, as can be seen in the confusion matrix created as part of the results for our random forest model, we can see that only "Long" survival can be predicted with high accuracy. This can be another reason behind the high error rates of the model. In several cases, we cannot observe a tight correlation between the independent and dependent variables, for all or certain of the classes in the data. Even though this can affect the overall accuracy of our model, the algorithms used and the predictive models created must not be blamed. It is important to remember that even the best predictive models cannot make accurate predictions if the correlation between the independent and dependent variables is loose. However, we can try different algorithms to find the one that results in the best accuracy.

As mentioned earlier, a higher number of trees (ntree) in the random forest usually results in better predictions. However, we mentioned that this improvement is not constant. If we plot (Fig. 11.1), our random forest model by

```
> plot(RF)
```

As can be seen, the error rates decrease with the increasing number of trees; however, in the case of our model, the lowest error rate is reached at 200 trees. We can opt to change the number of trees by changing the "ntree" parameter in our randomForest function. However, we move forward with the default number of trees.

Random forests can also be used for choosing the variables most predictive of the dependent variable in a data set. Remember that the decision tree from Chapter 12 suggested that the "Ki67 index" was the variable that could determine the survival time of patients. Random forests can help us understand the importance of each variable in determining the class of data points. In order to understand the importance of each feature, the decrease in the Gini index is calculated. The variable with the highest mean decrease in the Gini index is considered to be the most important variable, and as the mean decrease in the Gini index decreases, so does the importance of the variable.

But what is Gini index? We remember from Chapter 12 that the ID3 algorithm uses the entropy and information gain to make the decision tree. We also remember that there were other algorithms to make decision trees. One of these algorithms was the classification and regression tree algorithm. This algorithm uses the Gini index to make the decision trees. Similar to the entropy, the Gini index ranges from 0 to 1 and determines the probability of a feature being classified incorrectly if selected randomly. The Gini index is calculated as

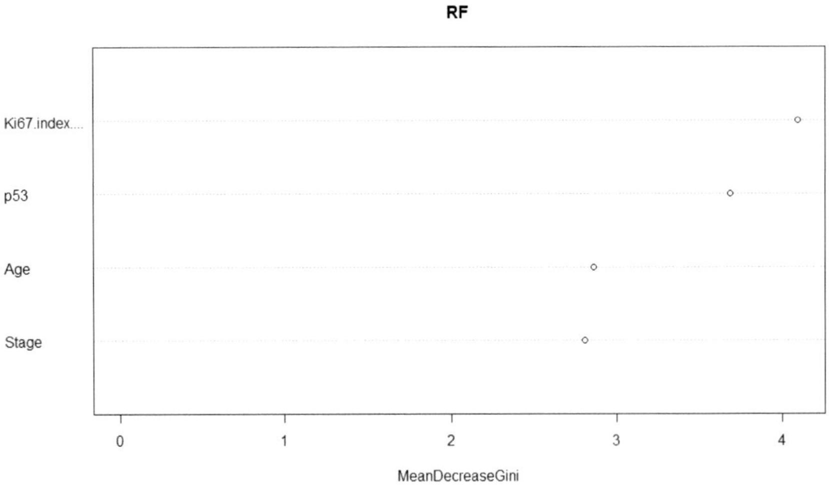

FIGURE 11.2 Plot of the importance of each variable based on the decrease in the Gini index.

follows:

$$G = 1 - \sum_{i=1}^{c} p_i^2. \tag{11.1}$$

Now, let us see the level of importance for each of the variables in our data set

```
> importance(RF)
                 MeanDecreaseGini
Age                      2.857474
Stage                    2.801020
Ki67.index....           4.088890
p53                      3.683593
```

The variable with the highest "mean decrease Gini" is the most important in determining the class. We can also use plots to understand the importance of each variable, which can be easier and more accelerated to retrieve information (Fig. 11.2)

```
> varImpPlot(RF)
```

Now, we need to test the accuracy of our model in predicting the testing subset classes. For this purpose, we create a confusion matrix using the "caret" package [6], which can provide more information compared to the confusion matrices made from R's built-in function table()

```
> library(caret)
> prediction <- predict(RF, test)
> confusionMatrix(prediction, test$Survival)
Confusion Matrix and Statistics

               Reference
Prediction      Intermediate Long Short
  Intermediate             1    1     0
  Long                     1    7     0
  Short                    1    0     2

Overall Statistics

               Accuracy : 0.7692
                 95% CI : (0.4619, 0.9496)
    No Information Rate : 0.6154
    P-Value [Acc > NIR] : 0.1986

                  Kappa : 0.5806

 Mcnemar's Test P-Value : NA

Statistics by Class:

                     Class: Intermediate Class: Long
Sensitivity                      0.33333      0.8750
Specificity                      0.90000      0.8000
Pos Pred Value                   0.50000      0.8750
Neg Pred Value                   0.81818      0.8000
Prevalence                       0.23077      0.6154
Detection Rate                   0.07692      0.5385
Detection Prevalence             0.15385      0.6154
Balanced Accuracy                0.61667      0.8375
                     Class: Short
Sensitivity                1.0000
Specificity                0.9091
Pos Pred Value             0.6667
Neg Pred Value             1.0000
Prevalence                 0.1538
Detection Rate             0.1538
Detection Prevalence       0.2308
Balanced Accuracy          0.9545
```

We can see that our overall accuracy has dramatically increased compared to the decision tree model from Chapter 12. Even though the accuracy is still not very high, the improvement in accuracy considering the sample size is proof of the better performance of random forest in predicting classes compared to decision trees. This improvement in prediction can be attributed to different decision trees taking into account different variables. In contrast to the decision tree created in Chapter 12, random forests are an ensemble of decision trees with various numbers of nodes and splitting patterns. We can get a better understanding of these features of the random forest by plotting the number of nodes in decision trees of the random forest (Fig. 11.3)

```
> hist(treesize(RF))
```

We can see that the number of nodes can increase to as high as 10 nodes, compared to the 3 nodes in the decision tree from Chapter 12. This results from considering various combinations of events and increases the accuracy of the model when faced with new data.

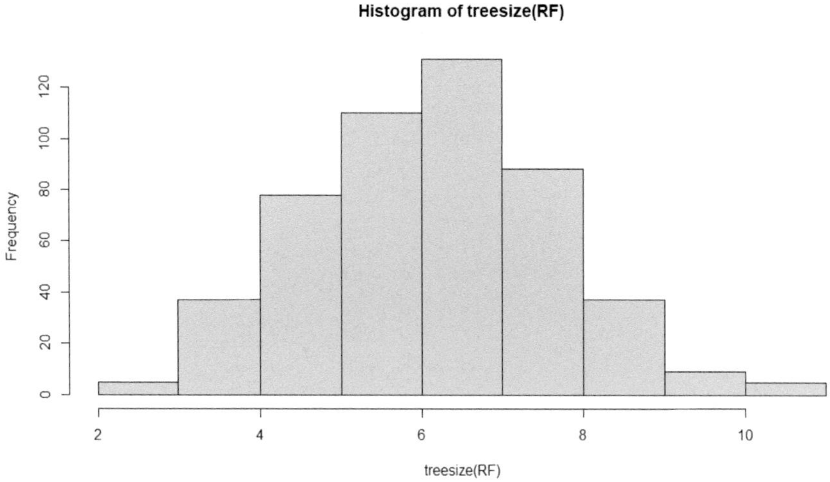

FIGURE 11.3 Number of nodes in decision trees created by the random forest algorithm.

Random forest regression

As mentioned earlier, random forests are also common regression algorithms. They do not have the restrictive assumptions of linear regression, which makes them useful for instances with nonlinearity in the data. Bootstrapping in random forests makes their predictions more reliable than other regression algorithms, including support vector regression [7]. In order to compare the performance of random forests with other regression algorithms learned thus far, we use the same data set used in the previous chapters to create regression models. Similar to previous chapters, we make sure that the structure of the data conforms to the nature of the variables and our predictive purposes

```
> str(reg_data)
'data.frame':   36 obs. of  5 variables:
 $ Age          : int  42 2 34 6 32 15 65 23 63 13 ...
 $ Stage        : int  3 1 2 2 2 4 2 4 3 2 ...
 $ Ki67.index....: int  78 12 46 63 83 80 15 78 51 46 ...
 $ p53          : int  6 0 2 11 23 28 1 13 0 1 ...
 $ Survival     : int  13 102 43 12 5 1 45 7 41 23 ...
> reg_data$Stage <- as.factor(reg_data$Stage)
```

We now divide our data set into training and testing subsets using the same dividing parameters used in previous chapters

```
> set.seed(123)
> subsets <- sample(2, nrow(reg_data), prob=c(0.7, 0.3), replace=T)
> reg_train <- reg_data[subsets==1,]
> reg_test <- reg_data[subsets==2,]
```

Now, our data are ready to train the random forest regression model. For regression models as well, we use the "randomForest" package and the randomForest() function from this package. The function will automatically return results for a regression problem as the output is a continuous variable. We will be creating two random forest regression models by changing certain parameters of the randomForest() function and evaluating their effect on the improvement of our model and the accuracy of our predictions

```
> reg_RF1 <- randomForest(Survival~., data=reg_train)
> reg_RF1

Call:
 randomForest(formula = Survival ~ ., data = reg_train)
               Type of random forest: regression
                     Number of trees: 500
No. of variables tried at each split: 1

          Mean of squared residuals: 362.4562
                    % Var explained: 48.75
```

The first few lines of the output when calling the model are similar to random forest classifiers as the number of trees generated to make predictions is by default set to 500. The mean of squared residuals is an indicator of how far our predictions are from the observed values and reflects the model's accuracy. Similar to other regression models, the smaller the mean of squared residuals, the better the accuracy of the model. "% Var explained" shows the percentage of variances in the observations that can be explained by our model. The higher this percentage is, the better our model can explain the observed data and the more accurate its predictions will be for unseen data.

There are several arguments in the randomForest() function that can be changed to improve the model's accuracy. One of these arguments is "importance," which when set to TRUE, will assess the importance of variables included in the model. We create a second regression model by setting this argument to TRUE and then we compare the two models in terms of the mean of squared residuals and other factors indicative of the model's accuracy, including root mean squared error (RMSE).

```
> reg_RF2 <- randomForest(Survival~., data=reg_train, importance=TRUE)
> reg_RF2

Call:
 randomForest(formula = Survival ~ ., data = reg_train, importance = TRUE)
               Type of random forest: regression
                     Number of trees: 500
No. of variables tried at each split: 1

          Mean of squared residuals: 324.3603
                    % Var explained: 54.13
```

As can be noted, the change of one argument has dramatically improved the models' parameters, indicative of its accuracy. Plotting these models gives us an idea of how the number of trees can affect models' accuracy, which can be helpful for changing other parameters of the model. Figs. 11.4 and 11.5 plot the reg_RF1 and reg_RF2 regression models, respectively. These plots will be useful to change the "ntree" argument of our models. By decreasing the number of trees, we can save prediction time for high-dimensional data sets.

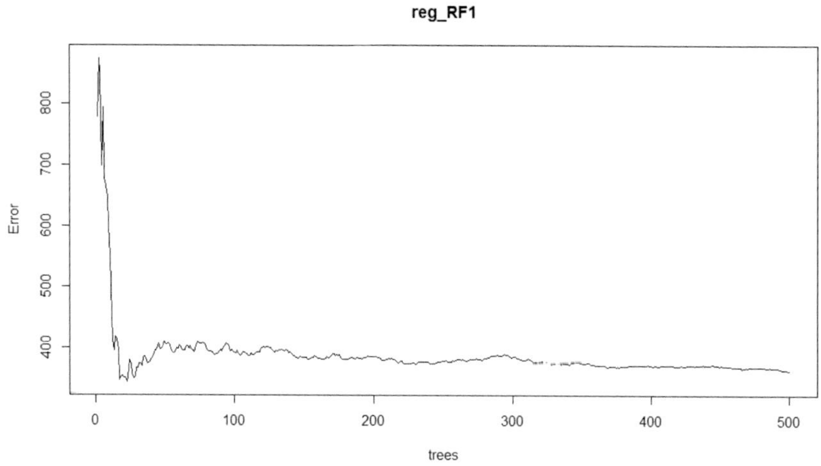

FIGURE 11.4 Plot of the reg_RF1 model. The error rate of the model remains virtually constant when the number of trees is above 150.

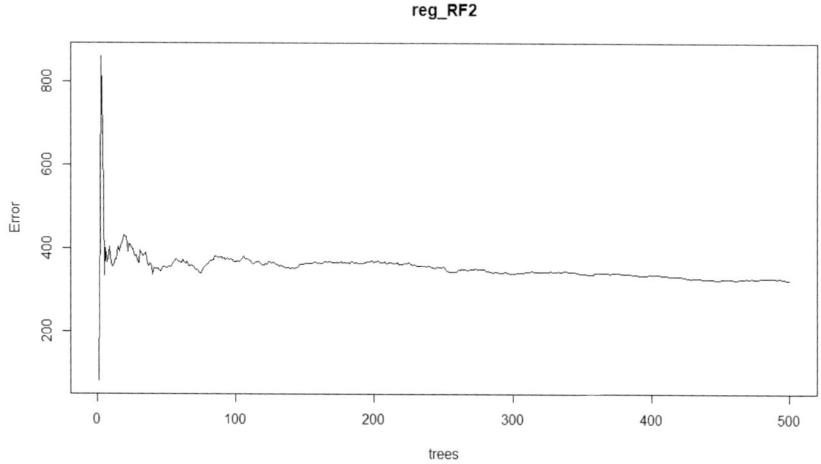

FIGURE 11.5 Plot of the reg_RF2 model. The error rate of the model remains virtually constant when the number of trees is above 100.

We now use the testing subset to understand the model's accuracy when predicting unseen data. For this purpose, we calculate the RMSE for both models and compare them to the RMSE of other regression models from previous chapters.

```
> library(Metrics)
> predict_RF1<- predict(reg_RF1, reg_test)
> RMSE_RF1 <- rmse(predict_RF1, reg_test$Survival)
> RMSE_RF1
[1] 12.57588

> predict_RF2<- predict(reg_RF2, reg_test)
> RMSE_RF2 <- rmse(predict_RF2, reg_test$Survival)
> RMSE_RF2
[1] 11.9732
```

Based on the RMSE values of the two models, we see that the change of "importance" argument can improve the predictive abilities of our models. We also see a dramatic improvement compared to other linear and nonlinear regression models, which can be attributed to the bootstrapping of our random forest regression model [7].

References

[1] K. Fawagreh, M.M. Gaber, E. Elyan, Random forests: from early developments to recent advancements, Systems Science & Control Engineering 2 (2014) 602–609.

[2] D. Denisko, M.M. Hoffman, Classification and interaction in random forests, Proceedings of the National Academy of Sciences of the United States of America 115 (8) (2018) 1690–1692.

[3] Q. Wang, T.T. Nguyen, J.Z. Huang, T.T. Nguyen, An efficient random forests algorithm for high dimensional data classification, Advances in Data Analysis and Classification 12 (2018) 953–972.

[4] T.T. Nguyen, J.Z. Huang, T.T. Nguyen, Unbiased feature selection in learning random forests for high-dimensional data, The Scientific World Journal 2015 (2015) 471371.

[5] A. Liaw, M. Wiener, Classification and regression by randomForest, R News 2 (3) (2002) 18–22.

[6] M. Kuhn, Caret package, Journal of Statistical Software 28 (5) (2008).

[7] B.F. Huang, P.C. Boutros, The parameter sensitivity of random forests, BMC Bioinformatics 17 (1) (2016) 331.

CHAPTER

12

K-nearest neighbors in R

What is K-nearest neighbors?

In previous chapters, we learned about supervised algorithms, most of which could be used for both classification and regression purposes. In this chapter, we will learn about another supervised algorithm, called K-nearest neighbors (KNN), last in the series of algorithms intended to be covered in this book. KNN can also be used for both regression and classification purposes [1]. The main purpose of using this algorithm in the classification and regression of unseen data in this algorithm is the output of the K-closest data points to the new, unseen data point [1]. The class of the majority of K-closest data points to a new data point, or the average of the K-closest data points, determines the class or value of the new data point in classification and regression problems, respectively.

The calculations behind KNN algorithms are relatively simple; however, it is computationally expensive. In order to determine the class or value of a data point, we need to find the distance between the new data point and other data points that have been used to train the algorithm. There are various methods to measure the distance of data points from one another [2]. Euclidean function is one of the most common methods used for this purpose. To find the distance between two points in a N-dimensional coordinate (N features) using the Euclidean function, we use the following formula:

$$d(i,j) = \sqrt{|x_{i1} - x_{j1}|^2 + |x_{i2} - x_{j2}|^2 + \cdots + |x_{in} - x_{jn}|^2} \tag{12.1}$$

After the distance between the data points with a known class or value and the new data point is calculated, data points are ranked based on their distances. We will then need to determine K to pick the first K-ranked data points to vote for the class or find the value of the new data set (Fig. 12.1). One of the most important steps in KNN is therefore determining the K, as

Immunoinformatics of Cancers
DOI: https://doi.org/10.1016/B978-0-12-822400-7.00006-3

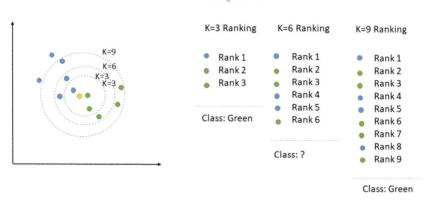

FIGURE 12.1 Implementing a KNN algorithm for finding the class of a new data point. The two classes in the training data are shown by blue and green dots. The new data point is shown by a yellow dot. The higher the number of KNN, the more accurate the classification of observations. *KNN*, K-nearest neighbors.

there is a tradeoff between model accuracy and its computational cost. It is evident that the higher the value of *K* is, the better the accuracy of the model will be as more data points are involved in voting for the class or value of the new data point (Fig. 12.1). Furthermore, a higher value for *K* allows more robustness regarding outliers. However, calculating the distance of the data points for higher values of *K* can be computationally costly. Even though there is no specific formula or shortcut to determining the value of *K*, there are certain approaches that suggest best possible values of *K*. One such approach is to set K as the square root of the number of data points in the training data set [3]. In addition, we can start off by assigning a random number to *K*, which is of course equal to or smaller than the number of data points used to train the model, and adjust the assigned value based on the output of the model. However, there are functions that test different values for *K*, and after cross-validation of data, they return the best values for *K*. We start off by assigning a random number to *K*, which is, of course, equal to or smaller than the number of data points used to train the model, and adjust the assigned value based on the output of the model.

KNN, being a nonparametric algorithm, has several advantages over parametric algorithms, which have assumptions regarding the data set. However, it is necessary to preprocess all independent variables before training the model as different scales of the features lead to disproportionate estimations of distances between the data points. There are various methods for standardizing data, all of which will be appropriate for preprocessing of data in KNN.

Another advantage of KNN is use of *K*-fold cross-validation by resampling subsets from the training data to train the model and test for model accuracy [4]. Use of cross-validation allows better training of the model in smaller data sets. In this method, the data are divided into K subsets, hence K-fold cross-validation. At each iteration, $K - 1$ subsets are used for training the data and 1 subset is spared for testing model accuracy. The number of iterations can be determined by the analyst, and the final accuracy of the model is the average of accuracies at each iteration [4].

Hands-on K-nearest neighbors in R

In this chapter, we will learn how to implement KNN for the prediction of categorical and continuous variables. In order to compare the performance of KNN with that of the algorithms discussed in previous chapters, we will use the data sets presented in Tables 9.1 and 9.3. We start off by learning how to implement KNN for classification problems.

For classification problems, similar to previous chapters, we need to ensure that the structure of the data set imported corresponds to the intended structure for the data set. Therefore, in the data set of neuroblastoma patients' survival from Table 9.3, we make sure that patients' stage of the disease and survival category are factor variables:

```
> str(data)
'data.frame':   36 obs. of  5 variables:
 $ Age          : int  42 2 34 6 32 15 65 23 63 13 ...
 $ Stage        : int  3 1 2 2 2 4 2 4 3 2 ...
 $ Ki67.index....: int  78 12 46 63 83 80 15 78 51 46 ...
 $ p53          : int  6 0 2 11 23 28 1 13 0 1 ...
 $ Survival     : chr  "Intermediate" "Long" "Long" "Long" ...
> data$Stage <- as.factor(data$Stage)
> data$Survival <- as.factor(data$Survival)
```

We need to standardize our data before dividing it into training and testing subsets. As mentioned earlier, there are different methods for standardizing data, some of which include normalizing with Z score so all variables will have values between −3 and 3, or using the min−max scaling method in which all variables are assigned values in a specific range, usually 0 and 1. There are certain build-in functions as well packages that can take care of standardizing the data. Two of the widely used methods for standardizing are "scale" and "center," which, in general, can implement the mentioned methods of standardization as arguments of the R built-in function `scale()`. However, some packages used for developing KNN models, such as the "caret" package [5], have preprocessing arguments. In this chapter, we will learn to train KNN models using the "caret" package; therefore no preprocessing is needed before dividing our data set into training and testing subsets. We use the same parameters as used in previous chapters to divide the data set into training and testing subsets so the results will be comparable between the different methods:

```
> set.seed(123)
> subsets <- sample(2, nrow(data), prob=c(0.7, 0.3), replace=T)
> train <- data[subsets==1,]
> test <- data[subsets==2,]
```

In order to train the KNN model, we use the "caret" package. In addition to standardizing the predictors, this package has the advantage of testing different values for *K* and returning values of *K* that minimize the errors in cross-validations and implementing the optimal *K* value to train the model.

```
> install.packages("caret")
> library(caret)
```

In order to train the KNN model, we use the `train()` function from the "caret" package. This function can be used for training models based on numerous algorithms, including but not limited to KNN, random forest, neural networks, linear regression, and discriminant analysis. This can be determined through the "method" argument of the train function. Another important argument of the `train()` function that needs to be determined when training models is "trControl" as this argument determines how the `train()` function acts to train the model. As mentioned earlier, the `train()` function of the "caret" package can preprocess the data. Another argument that needs to be determined by the analyst is "tuneLength." In KNN, this argument determines how many values for *K* should be tested in training the model. Evidently, the higher the number of *K* values tested, the better the chances of reaching a higher accuracy. However, the pace-limiting factor of computation, especially for high-dimensional data, must also be considered when choosing the number of values for *K* to be tested. Considering these parameters, we train the KNN model using the `train()` function from the "caret" package as given below:

```
> set.seed(1234)
> KNN <- train(Survival~., data=train,
+              method="knn",
+              trControl=trainControl("cv", number=5),
+              preProcess=c("scale", "center"),
+              tuneLength=25)
```

In order to understand how different *K* values can affect the accuracy of the model, we can plot the data (Fig. 12.2). Given the values tested, a value slightly smaller than 10 results in the highest accuracy (of almost 70%) for our model.

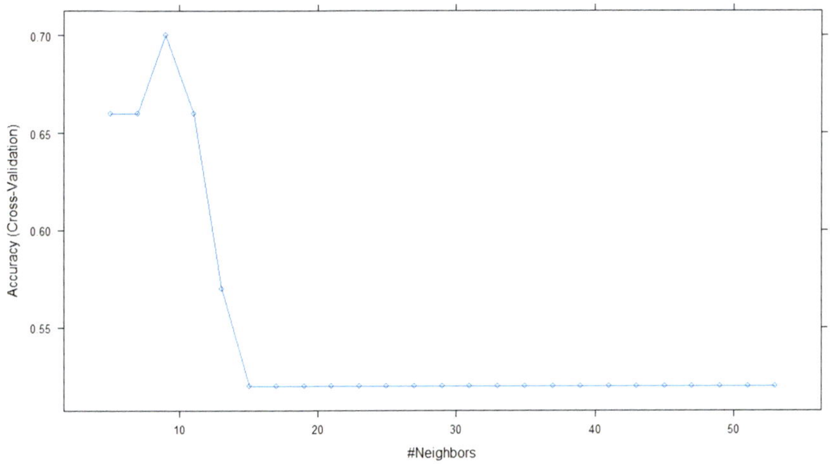

FIGURE 12.2 Plot of the KNN model. The accuracy of model is highest at $K = 9$, and does not change after $K = 15$. *KNN*, K-nearest neighbors.

```
> plot(KNN)
```

Furthermore, we can determine the best value for K by calling "bestTune" from the output of the model:

```
> KNN$bestTune
  k
3 9
```

NOTE...

When determining parameters for training a KNN model, there are certain points to be considered. The values assigned to the "tuneLength" argument need to be greater than 1. Furthermore, when training a KNN model, if the values that are being tested by the function `train()` are greater than the number of observations in the training data, the function will return *warnings*, which will not interfere with the performance of the function.

This shows that after trying different values for K, the third value tested, which was $K = 9$, resulted in the best accuracy for the model.

In order to compare the accuracy of the model with other supervised classification algorithms from previous chapters, we predict the class of observations in the testing subset using our model. In order to get the confusion matrix for our predictions, we use the `ConfusionMatrix()` function from the "caret" package:

```
> prediction <- predict(KNN, test)
> confusionMatrix(prediction, test$Survival)
Confusion Matrix and Statistics

              Reference
Prediction     Intermediate Long Short
  Intermediate            1    1     1
  Long                    1    7     0
  Short                   1    0     1

Overall Statistics

               Accuracy : 0.6923
                 95% CI : (0.3857, 0.9091)
    No Information Rate : 0.6154
    P-Value [Acc > NIR] : 0.3966

                  Kappa : 0.4348

 Mcnemar's Test P-Value : NA

Statistics by Class:

                     Class: Intermediate Class: Long
Sensitivity                      0.33333      0.8750
Specificity                      0.80000      0.8000
Pos Pred Value                   0.33333      0.8750
Neg Pred Value                   0.80000      0.8000
Prevalence                       0.23077      0.6154
Detection Rate                   0.07692      0.5385
Detection Prevalence             0.23077      0.6154
Balanced Accuracy                0.56667      0.8375
                     Class: Short
Sensitivity               0.50000
Specificity               0.90909
Pos Pred Value            0.50000
Neg Pred Value            0.90909
Prevalence                0.15385
Detection Rate            0.07692
Detection Prevalence      0.15385
Balanced Accuracy         0.70455
```

Like previous chapters, best predictions belong to the "Long" survival category, as the number of observations belonging to the "Long" category is more than the other two classes in the test subset:

```
> sum(test$Survival=="Long")
[1] 8
> sum(test$Survival=="Short")
[1] 2
> sum(test$Survival=="Intermediate")
[1] 3
```

A brief overview of the rest of the `ConfusionMatrix()` output shows an overall accuracy of 0.69, which considering the sample size is considerable. The "no information rate" is the largest class percentage in data, which belongs to the class "Long" survival, which holds 8 observations out of the total 13 observations in the testing subset (61%). This imbalance in proportions of the observation classes can lead to misinterpretation of model accuracy, as the model is biased to report more observations as the class with highest proportion in testing data. In order to understand whether our model has better accuracy over merely assigning classes based on class proportions, we need to see if the *P*-value of the model denotes significantly better accuracy over assigning classes randomly based on class proportions. In other words, is the 69% overall accuracy really better than the 61% of the largest class proportion? The *P*-value of our model denies such supremacy of the model over "no information rate," with *P*-value [Acc > NIR] > 0.05. Therefore, despite a considerable overall accuracy percentage, this accuracy cannot be attributed to the model. Another parameter of the `ConfusionMatrix()` output is the Kappa coefficient, which ranges between −1 and 1. A Kappa of 1 shows highest model accuracy compared with a random model, and a Kappa of −1 shows the lowest level of accuracy compared with a random model. A Kappa of 0 shows that the accuracy of the developed model is as good as the map or a random model. Therefore a Kappa coefficient of 0.43 confirms that the model's accuracy is slightly better than a random model, which combined with the *P*-value of the model shows this improvement is random and due to class proportion imbalance. Since there are more than two classes in our target variables, McNemar's test, which determines whether there is a difference in a dichotomous dependent variable between two related groups, is therefore not applicable for our data set.

A comparison of the KNN with previous classification models introduced in this book shows that the accuracy of this model is not the best. The factors discussed in this chapter and previous chapters must be considered when choosing the optimal classification algorithm for our model. For the specific data set we used for classification in this book, one of the algorithms was random forests due to its bootstrapping. Even though a similar method is used in KNN in terms of resampling, the methods for similarity finding of random forests work better with our data set.

Now we compare the performance of KNN with models from previous chapters for regression problems, using the same data set, called reg_data here.

```
> str(reg_data)
'data.frame':   36 obs. of  5 variables:
 $ Age            : int  42 2 34 6 32 15 65 23 63 13 ...
 $ Stage          : int  3 1 2 2 2 4 2 4 3 2 ...
 $ Ki67.index....: int  78 12 46 63 83 80 15 78 51 46 ...
 $ p53            : int  6 0 2 11 23 28 1 13 0 1 ...
 $ Survival       : int  13 102 43 12 5 1 45 7 41 23 ...
```

We need to change the structure of the data set in order for all variables to conform to their nature based on our background knowledge. Therefore we change the class of the "Stage" variable from integer to factor:

```
> reg_data$Stage <- as.factor(reg_data$Stage)
```

Now our data set is ready to be divided into training and testing subsets. As we need to compare the performance of the KNN in regression problems with other regression models, we use the same parameters for dividing the data set into training and testing subsets that we used in previous chapters:

```
> set.seed(123)
> subsets <- sample(2, nrow(reg_data), prob=c(0.7, 0.3), replace=T)
> reg_train <- reg_data[subsets==1,]
> reg_test <- reg_data[subsets==2,]
```

The steps for training a KNN model for regression are very similar to the steps used for creating KNN models for classification problems. We use the same function from the "caret" package to train the model based on the training data:

```
> reg_KNN <- train(Survival~., data=reg_train,
+                  method="knn",
+                  trControl=trainControl("cv", number=5),
+                  preProcess=c("center", "scale"),
+                  tuneLength=25)
```

Even though the steps for training the regression model were similar to the steps for training a KNN classifier, the outcome is the opposite of that of the classifiers. In classification, we are looking for values of *K* that result in the highest accuracy; therefore we look for the *K* that results in the global maximum value in the plot. However, in a KNN regression model, we look for values of *K* that return the lowest root mean squared error (RMSE). In order to find such values for *K*, we can either plot the model (Fig. 12.3) or call the "bestTune" parameter of the model to find the exact *K* to return lowest RMSE:

```
> plot(reg_KNN)
> reg_KNN$bestTune
  k
1 5
```

We now know that $K = 5$ results in the lowest RMSE. The model will use this *K* for making further predictions. In order to find the performance of the model when faced with new data, we use the reg_KNN model to predict the values for the testing subset. We use the `rmse()` function from the "Metrics" package [6]:

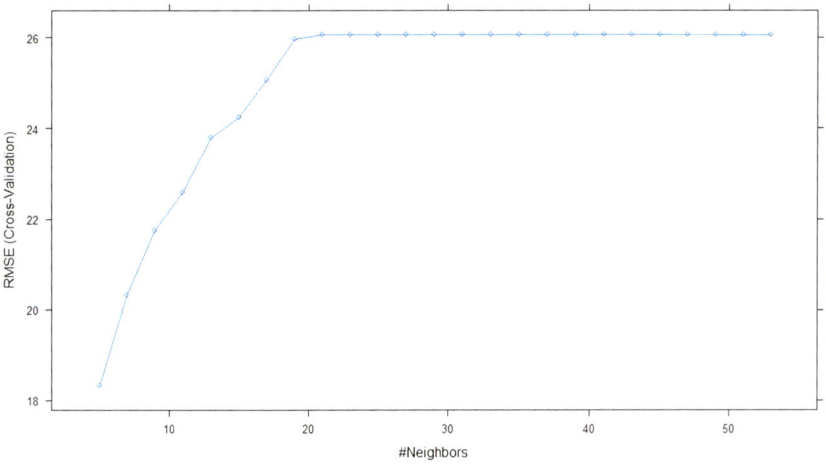

FIGURE 12.3 Plot of the KNN regression model. #Neighbors shows the *K* values tested by the model. The *K* value that returns the lowest RMSE is the best value for *K* to tune the model. *KNN*, K-nearest neighbors; *RMSE*, root mean squared error.

```
> library(Metrics)
> reg_predict <- predict(reg_KNN, reg_test)
> RMSE_KNN <- rmse(reg_predict, reg_test$Survival)
> RMSE_KNN
[1] 14.77695
```

A comparison of the RMSE from a KNN model with that of the regression models created in previous chapters shows better performance compared to the parametric models such as linear regression; however, the performance of some other nonparametric algorithms such as random forest is better than that of the KNN. The small size of the training data is one of the reasons behind better performance of random forests over KNN; however, random forests handle large data sets well, too.

A general key to developing a good predictive model, whether it is a regression model or a classification model, is to have an understanding regarding the structure of the data and the relationship between the variables in the data set and the different parameters when training a model. These concepts will be revisited in Chapter 14 through practical examples.

References

[1] Z. Zhang, Introduction to machine learning: k-nearest neighbors, Annals of Translational Medicine 4 (11) (2016) 218. Available from: https://doi.org/10.21037/atm.2016.03.37.

[2] L.Y. Hu, M.W. Huang, S.W. Ke, C.F. Tsai, The distance function effect on k-nearest neighbor classification for medical datasets, SpringerPlus 5 (1) (2016) 1304. Available from: https://doi.org/10.1186/s40064-016-2941-7.

[3] H. Raeisi Shahraki, S. Pourahmad, N. Zare, *K* important neighbors: a novel approach to binary classification in high dimensional data, BioMed Research International 2017 (2017) 7560807. Available from: https://doi.org/10.1155/2017/7560807.

[4] M.A. Little, G. Varoquaux, S. Saeb, L. Lonini, A. Jayaraman, D.C. Mohr, et al., Using and understanding cross-validation strategies. Perspectives on Saeb et al, GigaScience 6 (5) (2017) 1–6. Available from: https://doi.org/10.1093/gigascience/gix020.

[5] M. Kuhn, Caret package, Journal of Statistical Software 28 (5) (2008).

[6] Hamner, B., Frasco, M., LeDell, E. (2018). Metrics: Evaluation Metrics for Machine Learning. An implementation of evaluation metrics in R that are commonly used in supervised machine learning. It implements metrics for regression, time series, binary classification, classification, and information retrieval problems. It has zero dependencies and a consistent, simple interface for all functions.

CHAPTER

13

Neural networks in R

What are neural networks?

Neural networks are complex machine learning algorithms whose mechanism of action and decision making is inspired by that of the nervous system [1]. These algorithms are considered as both supervised learning algorithms and unsupervised learning algorithms, based on their use [2]. These algorithms can be used both for classification and regression, as well as for clustering through unsupervised learning [1]. We encounter examples of neural networks in today's world on a daily basis. Face recognition by smart phones, estimated time of arrival and choice of best routes by navigation applications, text-to-speech algorithms, and natural language processing are a few examples where neural networks are in use. Use of neural networks in medicine is becoming more and more profound, with algorithms helping with decision making and diagnosis, especially through image processing and natural language processing [3]. Furthermore, these algorithms can be used to simulate or discover new patterns in biological data [4,5]. Cancer research is another field of medicine that is benefiting from neural networks, alongside other machine learning algorithms [6,7]. Advances in both computer sciences and high-throughput technology have resulted in high-dimension data that require complex algorithms to be interpreted. Neural networks can be used both for dimensionality reduction through clustering, and for classification and regression problems in multiomics data [6,7]. The use of neural networks and the algorithms used in bioinformatics is beyond the scope of this book. Therefore we provide a brief introduction to some of the neural network algorithms and their application in bioinformatics. In this chapter, we focus on the supervised neural networks for classification and regression problems, as well as self-organizing maps (SOMs), one of the most common unsupervised neural networks algorithms.

Immunoinformatics of Cancers
DOI: https://doi.org/10.1016/B978-0-12-822400-7.00014-2

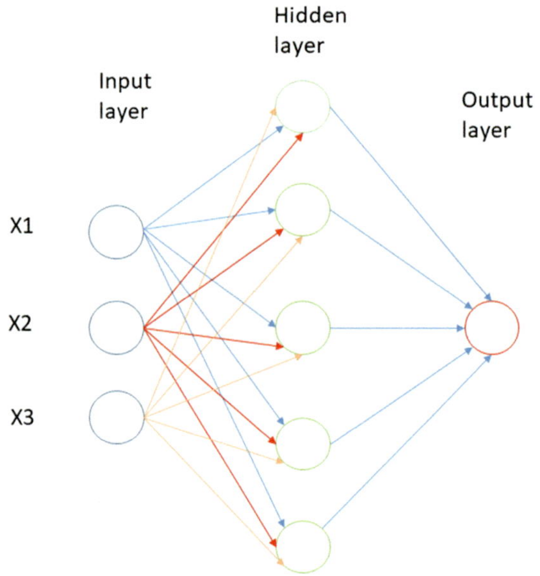

FIGURE 13.1 Schematic diagram of artificial neural networks composed of an input layer with three nodes (neurons), a hidden layers with five neurons, and an output layer with the output node. Depending on the algorithms used, the output layer can be composed of one or more neurons.

Neural networks resemble the nervous system in that they are composed of different layers, and the output from each layer acts as an input for the consecutive layers [1]. Each neural network is composed of at least three layers: an input layer, a hidden layer, and an output layer. The hidden layer can be composed of one or several layers, depending on how complex the neural network is (Fig. 13.1).

In each layer, there can be different numbers of nodes, or neurons. For the input layer, the number of the neurons is determined by the number of the features in the training data, and for each feature, a node is present. Most neural network models also include an extra node in this layer, for the bias term, which will be discussed later. The number of nodes in the output layer depends on whether the model is solving a regression problem, meaning the output is a numeric value, or whether it is handling a classification problem, where the outputs are classes. For regression problems, the output layer will have only one node. If the neural network deals with a classification problem, the output layer usually has one neuron; however, depending on the functions used to create the neural networks, the number of neurons in the output layer can be equal to the number of possible classes of the target variable [8].

The decision regarding the number of layers and neurons to be used in each layer of the hidden layers depends on the nature of the data set, and how complex the neural networks need to be in order to make accurate decisions [8]. Another aspect to be considered while determining the number of layers and neurons in a neural network is whether a neural network is required for making predictions in our data. Even though neural networks are among the most accurate models to make predictions, it must be remembered that this accuracy is at the expense of the model's complexity, which may prove costly in terms of number of computations and required time to make predictions [8]. Therefore, if a data set is linearly separable, other predictive models such as linear regressions, support vector machines, and other parametric models discussed in previous chapters might be more efficient for making predictions, which is similar to a neural network with no hidden layers [9,10].

Following up on the concept of simplicity of predictive models, the number of hidden layers must not be increased unless required to increase the model's accuracy dramatically. In most models, one hidden layer is sufficient for making accurate predictions, and an addition of more hidden layers is not likely to improve the performance of the model dramatically. Even though there are various methods to determine the number of neurons in the hidden layer, a good rule of thumb to determine the number of neurons is the average of the input and output neurons. However, this number can be further adjusted in optimizing and tuning steps in order to improve the accuracy of the model.

Now that the general structure of a neural network has been discussed, let us briefly overview the calculations behind decision making in neural networks. There are various forms of neural networks, including but not limited to feedforward neural networks, convolutional neural networks, and recurrent neural networks. We focus on details of feedforward neural networks, which are among the first and most applied neural networks in bioinformatics. A closer look at Fig. 13.1 reveals that there are several arrows coming out of each node in the input layer, and the number of arrows is determined by the number of nodes in the next layer, which is the hidden layer. The same holds true for each node in the hidden layers, which feed input for nodes in the next layer of the hidden layer, or the output layer through arrows. Each of these arrows has an assigned weight, which determines the importance of its corresponding node in predicting the outcome: The higher the weight assigned to these nodes and arrows is, the more important they will be in deciding the output class or value [8].

Each node in the hidden layer has a threshold of activation or firing, which resembles transfer of signals in the nervous system. If the sum of the inputs to each node surpasses the activation threshold, the node is activated and transfers signal to nodes to the next level through its weighted arrow. The sum of inputs to each node is calculated by summing the product of weights of nodes and arrows received by the node, plus a bias parameter, which, similar to a bias or an intercept in other learning algorithms such as linear regression, is added to the input to adjust it [8].

$$\text{Input} = f(x) = \sum_{i=1}^{m} w_i x_i + \text{bias} = w_1 x_1 + w_2 x_2 + \ldots + w_m x_m + \text{bias} \tag{13.1}$$

where w is the weight assigned to the node and x is the value of the node. Based on the activation functions implemented in the model, this input from other nodes, which in a feedforward model is received from the previous node, will determine whether the corresponding node is activated, and if so, it will pass the product of its input and its weight to the next node. The type of activation function greatly impacts how neural networks make predictions [11]. One of the simpler forms of the activation function is the binary activation function.

$$\text{Output} = \begin{cases} 1 & if \quad f(x) > \text{threshold} \\ 0 & if \quad f(x) < \text{threshold} \end{cases} \tag{13.2}$$

When this function is implemented in neural networks, each neuron is called a perceptron. In such neural networks, if the sum of the inputs and bias received by a perceptron is greater than the activation threshold for the perceptron, the perceptron is activated and passes its output to the next perceptron [1]. In such neural networks, a slight change in each of the input values can create dramatic changes in the results. Therefore later models developed implemented other activation functions that moderate the impact of changes in values received by each neuron. There are several activation functions developed, with each neural network developed for a specific task [11]. The aim of such activation functions was to increase the accuracy of the model by better reflecting the role of each variable and each node in the final output of the model. One such activation function is the Rectified Linear Unit. This activation function better reflects values of different variables and inputs once the sum of the inputs to the node is greater than the activation threshold:

$$\text{Output} = \begin{cases} x & if \quad f(x) > \text{threshold} \\ 0 & if \quad f(x) < \text{threshold} \end{cases} \tag{13.3}$$

Even though this activation threshold better reflects the impact of each variable, this reflection only works one way for inputs greater than the threshold. Another activation function that better moderates role of variables is the sigmoid or logistic activation function:

$$\text{Output} = f(x) = \frac{1}{1 + e^{-x}} \tag{13.4}$$

This function is more commonly used for classification neural networks [11]. The output of the sigmoid function is a probability, and if this probability is greater than the probability predetermined for that node, the node is considered in the final output of the model. Since the output values in a sigmoid function range between 0 and 1, the threshold is usually considered 0.5; however, this threshold can be changed by the analyst based on the nature of the model, like any other logistic model.

In addition to the weights assigned to each node, and the thresholds for activation for nodes, another important factor that determines the performance and accuracy of the model is the cost function [12]. Similar to other predictive models, the cost function determines how much deviation exists between the actual value or class of observations and the predicted outcome, and the aim is to find parameters for the model that will result in the least deviation possible.

$$\text{Cost function} = \frac{\sum_{i=1}^{m}(\hat{y}_i - y_i)}{m} \tag{13.5}$$

where $\hat{y}$ is the predicted value and y is the actual value of the observation. In order to minimize the cost function, we try to find parameters that will result in the lowest gradient of the cost function, a process known as gradient decent [12]. In this process, random weights primarily assigned to each node are changed after the introduction of each node and variable to the model at each iteration, trying to reach the local minimum of the cost function. There are several ways of improving the model's predictions. In a feedforward model, backpropagation is one of the common methods used to improve the model's performance. In this method, in order to tune the weight of nodes to find the minimum value of the cost function, we adjust the weights by moving from the output layer toward the input layer, a process known as backpropagation, details of which is beyond the scope of this chapter [13].

Neural networks can have advantages over other learning algorithms. For instance, neural networks can better capture and reflect complexities between the variables in the data set, lower the risk of overfitting, and better handle high-dimensional data, which are due to the many parameters involved in the learning of the neural networks [1]. However, neural networks have their own limitations, like any other learning algorithm. Unlike several algorithms such as decision trees, random forests, and K-nearest neighbors that allow variables to be either numeric or categorical classes, neural networks cannot handle categorical variables, and in order to include categorical variables, these variables need to be preprocessed before being used to train the data [1]. There are a few ways of solving the categorical problems, including but not limited to dummy coding, one-hot encoding, and embedding, the latter being helpful especially when there are several possible classes for the variables for which there is no specific order or relationship. In this chapter, we will cover one-hot encoding, which is one of the most common ways of handling categorical variables. In this method, each class of a categorical variable will be fed to the neural network as a variable. As an example, consider the family history of cancer being a categorical variable for predicting the risk of developing cancer, and "first-degree," "second-degree," and "absent" being the three possible classes for this variable (Table 13.1). In order to feed this as an input to our neural network using one-hot encoding, each of these classes will become a separate binary variable when training the model (Table 13.2).

TABLE 13.1 Categorical variable before one-hot encoding.

Patient	Family history of cancer
A	Absent
B	First degree
C	Second degree
D	Second degree
E	Absent

TABLE 13.2 Categorical variable after one-hot encoding.

Patient	Family history of cancer—absent	Family history of cancer—first degree	Family history of cancer—second degree
A	1	0	0
B	0	1	0
C	0	0	1
D	0	0	1
E	1	0	0

Another aspect to be borne in mind when training neural networks is that the data need to be standardized before being used to train neural networks. This is because each variable is assigned a weight, and if data are not standardized before training the models, the weights assigned to nodes will be affected by their magnitude, which can be only reflective of differences in nature of variables.

Hands-on neural networks in R

We took a rather simplistic look at computations behind neural networks and learned about some of their advantages and limitations. In order to compare their performance with other learning algorithms, which can be considered "more conventional" for simpler data sets, we use the same data sets used in previous chapters to create classification and regression neural networks.

In order to better capture effects of model complexity and data preprocessing on the outcome of the model, we will develop several neural networks in this chapter using the same data set and compare their results.

We start by making the classification models. Our data set for classification models includes both numeric and categorical variables, the categorical variable being the stage of the cancer, with four possible levels of "1," "2," "3," and "4." In previous chapters, we transformed the class of this variable to make it a factor variable to reflect the nature of the variable. In this chapter, we will do the same to train one of the classification models in order to demonstrate one-hot encoding, in addition to comparing the results with another classification model in which this variable will not be transformed. We will also increase the complexity of neural networks by adding the number of hidden layers to understand the advantages and disadvantages of increasing model complexity.

For the first classification model, we do not convert the "Stage" variable. The reason for keeping the variable as numeric is that the order of the numbers reflects the nature of this variable. However, we still require standardizing our data set. We call this neural network model NN1. We start by checking the structure of the data, and for NN1, we keep the "Stage" as numeric, but we still need to change the dependent variable to a factor variable:

```
> str(data)
'data.frame':   36 obs. of  5 variables:
 $ Age          : int  42 2 34 6 32 15 65 23 63 13 ...
 $ Stage        : int  3 1 2 2 2 4 2 4 3 2 ...
 $ Ki67.index....: int  78 12 46 63 83 80 15 78 51 46 ...
 $ p53          : int  6 0 2 11 23 28 1 13 0 1 ...

 $ Survival     : chr  "Intermediate" "Long" "Long" "Long" ...
> data$Survival <- as.factor(data$Survival)
```

NOTE

As was mentioned earlier, neural networks start by assigning random weights to different neurons, and at each iteration, they modify these weights to minimize the error of the model. Therefore the results obtained from training models by even using the parameters can be different due to the effect of randomizations occurring at assigning weights, or the order in which features and observations are introduced to the model. To ensure reproducibility of results, it is important to prevent effects of randomization through the set.seed() function.

As mentioned earlier, we need to preprocess our data set by standardizing numeric variables of the data set. For this purpose, we use the built-in R function scale(). This function only takes numeric variables; therefore we must make sure that categorical variables are excluded:

```
> data[,-5] <- scale(data[,-5], center = T, scale = T)
> head(data)
          Age      Stage Ki67.index....        p53     Survival
1  0.45661482  0.6272964     1.30112277 -0.2976903 Intermediate
2 -1.26016153 -1.3364141    -1.32991357 -0.9745440         Long
3  0.11325955 -0.3545589     0.02546879 -0.7489261         Long
4 -1.08848389 -0.3545589     0.70315996  0.2663545         Long
5  0.02742073 -0.3545589     1.50044370  1.6200618        Short
6 -0.70220921  1.6091517     1.38085114  2.1841066        Short
```

We can now divide our data set into training and testing subsets. For comparison with previous classification models, we use the same parameters used in previous chapters:

```
> set.seed(123)
> subsets <- sample(2, nrow(data), prob=c(0.7, 0.3), replace=T)
> train <- data[subsets==1,]
> test <- data[subsets==2,]
```

We can now train our neural networks. There are several packages that can be used to create neural network models in R. One of the most widely used packages for this purpose is the "neuralnet" package [14].

```
> install.packages("neuralnet")
> library(neuralnet)
```

In order to train the model, we use the neuralnet() function from the "neuralnet" package.

```
> set.seed(123)
NN1 <- neuralnet(Survival~., data=train,
                 hidden=3, act.fct = "logistic",
                 linear.output = F, err.fct="ce", threshold = 0.01)
```

Similar to other model training functions, this function also has several arguments determining the parameters used to train the model. Some of these parameters are essential to be determined, such as the number of hidden neurons or the type of activation function to be used. In our model, we chose three nodes to be included in our hidden layer (hidden = 3), and chose the sigmoid or logistic function as our activation function for training the data (act.fct = "logistic"). For our error function, which calculates the deviation of the model's prediction for the training data set from their actual value, we chose cross-entropy over sum of squared errors (err.fct = "ce"). We set the threshold to 0.01, which determines the threshold for the derivative of the error function that we aim to reach, and until that threshold is not reached by the model, the model is not finalized in terms of correcting weights of neurons. It is preferable to avoid setting contrasting arguments for the model, such as threshold and the maximum number of steps allowed for neural networks.

Details of each neural network model can be found by using the summary() or print() function, or by simply calling the model:

```
> NN1
$call
neuralnet(formula = Survival ~ ., data = train, hidden = 3, threshold = 0.01,
    err.fct = "ce", act.fct = "logistic", linear.output = F)

$response
   Intermediate  Long Short
1          TRUE FALSE FALSE
2         FALSE  TRUE FALSE
3         FALSE FALSE  TRUE
4         FALSE  TRUE FALSE
5         FALSE  TRUE FALSE
6          TRUE FALSE FALSE
7         FALSE  TRUE FALSE
8          TRUE FALSE FALSE
9         FALSE FALSE  TRUE
10         TRUE FALSE FALSE
11        FALSE  TRUE FALSE
12        FALSE FALSE  TRUE
```

```
13        FALSE  TRUE FALSE
14        FALSE  TRUE FALSE
15        FALSE FALSE  TRUE
16        FALSE  TRUE FALSE
17         TRUE FALSE FALSE
18        FALSE FALSE  TRUE
19        FALSE  TRUE FALSE
20        FALSE  TRUE FALSE
21        FALSE  TRUE FALSE
22        FALSE  TRUE FALSE
23        FALSE FALSE  TRUE

$covariate
          Age      Stage Ki67.index....        p53
1   0.4566148  0.6272964     1.30112277 -0.2976903
3   0.1132596 -0.3545589     0.02546879 -0.7489261
6  -0.7022092  1.6091517     1.38085114  2.1841066
7   1.4437612 -0.3545589    -1.21032101 -0.8617350
9   1.3579224  0.6272964     0.22478972 -0.9745440
10 -0.7880480 -0.3545589     0.02546879 -0.8617350
12  0.9716477 -0.3545589     0.50383903  0.2663545
13  1.7441971  1.6091517    -0.25358052  0.4919724
14 -1.2172421  0.6272964     1.02207346  1.9584887
15 -0.7451286  0.6272964     0.66329578  1.3944439
17 -1.2601615 -1.3364141    -0.01439540 -0.5233082
18  0.4995342  1.6091517     0.50383903  1.6200618
19 -0.6592898 -0.3545589    -1.25018519 -0.8617350
22 -0.6163704 -0.3545589    -0.89140751 -0.9745440
23 -0.2300957 -0.3545589     1.73962882 -0.9745440
25 -1.3030809 -1.3364141    -1.40964194 -0.9745440
27  1.7012777  0.6272964    -0.17385215 -0.7489261
28 -1.1743227  1.6091517     1.30112277  1.3944439
29 -0.7022092 -0.3545589    -0.89140751  0.2663545
30  1.5296000 -1.3364141    -1.21032101 -0.5233082
33 -0.6163704 -0.3545589    -0.89140751 -0.9745440
35  0.2420178 -1.3364141    -1.36977776 -0.9745440
36 -0.8309674  0.6272964    -0.25358052  0.3791634

$model.list
$model.list$response
[1] "Intermediate" "Long"         "Short"

$model.list$variables
[1] "Age"              "Stage"            "Ki67.index...." "p53"


$err.fct
function (x, y)
{
    -(y * log(x) + (1 - y) * log(1 - x))
}
<bytecode: 0x000001dd0aa2e5d0>
<environment: 0x000001dd1c9f17c0>
attr(,"type")
[1] "ce"

$act.fct
function (x)
{
    1/(1 + exp(-x))
}
<bytecode: 0x000001dd0aa72570>
<environment: 0x000001dd1c47f030>
attr(,"type")
[1] "logistic"

$linear.output
[1] FALSE
```

```
$data
          Age      Stage Ki67.index....        p53     Survival
1   0.4566148  0.6272964    1.30112277 -0.2976903 Intermediate
3   0.1132596 -0.3545589    0.02546879 -0.7489261         Long
6  -0.7022092  1.6091517    1.38085114  2.1841066        Short
7   1.4437612 -0.3545589   -1.21032101 -0.8617350         Long
9   1.3579224  0.6272964    0.22478972 -0.9745440         Long
10 -0.7880480 -0.3545589    0.02546879 -0.8617350 Intermediate
12  0.9716477 -0.3545589    0.50383903  0.2663545         Long
13  1.7441971  1.6091517   -0.25358052  0.4919724 Intermediate
14 -1.2172421  0.6272964    1.02207346  1.9584887        Short
15 -0.7451286  0.6272964    0.66329578  1.3944439 Intermediate
17 -1.2601615 -1.3364141   -0.01439540 -0.5233082         Long
18  0.4995342  1.6091517    0.50383903  1.6200618        Short
19 -0.6592898 -0.3545589   -1.25018519 -0.8617350         Long
22 -0.6163704 -0.3545589   -0.89140751 -0.9745440         Long
23 -0.2300957 -0.3545589    1.73962882 -0.9745440        Short
25 -1.3030809 -1.3364141   -1.40964194 -0.9745440         Long
27  1.7012777  0.6272964   -0.17385215 -0.7489261 Intermediate
28 -1.1743227  1.6091517    1.30112277  1.3944439        Short
29 -0.7022092 -0.3545589   -0.89140751  0.2663545         Long
30  1.5296000 -1.3364141   -1.21032101 -0.5233082         Long
33 -0.6163704 -0.3545589   -0.89140751 -0.9745440         Long
35  0.2420178 -1.3364141   -1.36977776 -0.9745440         Long
36 -0.8309674  0.6272964   -0.25358052  0.3791634        Short

$exclude
NULL

$net.result
$net.result[[1]]
           [,1]         [,2]         [,3]
1  9.999768e-01 0.000000e+00 2.172172e-04
3  7.961210e-08 1.000000e+00 0.000000e+00
6  1.742211e-01 0.000000e+00 1.000000e+00
7  3.691106e-08 1.000000e+00 0.000000e+00
9  4.962654e-01 4.933661e-01 2.553334e-04
10 9.999515e-01 0.000000e+00 3.143156e-87
12 3.701936e-08 1.000000e+00 0.000000e+00
13 9.999768e-01 0.000000e+00 1.220925e-04
14 1.602805e-01 0.000000e+00 9.848665e-01
15 1.560900e-01 0.000000e+00 1.854047e-02
17 3.691270e-08 1.000000e+00 0.000000e+00
18 1.741645e-01 0.000000e+00 1.000000e+00
19 7.509539e-03 9.978617e-01 0.000000e+00
22 7.875522e-03 9.977279e-01 0.000000e+00
23 6.231866e-06 5.343054e-08 1.000000e+00
25 3.691085e-08 1.000000e+00 0.000000e+00
27 4.805360e-01 5.133138e-01 2.143057e-11
28 1.742212e-01 0.000000e+00 1.000000e+00
29 3.721238e-08 1.000000e+00 0.000000e+00
30 3.691085e-08 1.000000e+00 0.000000e+00
33 7.875522e-03 9.977279e-01 0.000000e+00
35 3.691085e-08 1.000000e+00 0.000000e+00
36 1.610167e-01 0.000000e+00 9.962738e-01
```

```
$weights
$weights[[1]]
$weights[[1]][[1]]
           [,1]       [,2]       [,3]
[1,]  -7.752387   2.012775  143.17611
[2,] -68.025580   2.957924   43.64644
[3,]  97.458016 -12.343329 -259.02368
[4,]  15.314982  -7.107448   36.17958
[5,]   3.786085   6.500512  267.66434

$weights[[1]][[2]]
            [,1]          [,2]          [,3]
[1,]  -0.01462353 -2.693631e-02    -8.1911571
[2,]  10.68718457 -1.233508e+03    -0.2430188
[3,]  -4.87157476  6.175252e+00 -1260.7866933
[4,] -12.22856207  1.298730e+01    38.5269374


$generalized.weights
$generalized.weights[[1]]
           [,1]          [,2]          [,3]          [,4]          [,5]
[,6]
1  -2.512043e-06 1.048269e-05 6.036041e-06 -5.520645e-06           NaN
NaN
3  -1.914894e+00 7.990796e+00 4.601204e+00 -4.208287e+00 2.427337e+00 -1.0129
20e+01
6  -2.560759e-06 1.068597e-05 6.153121e-06 -5.627680e-06           NaN
NaN
7  -1.685929e-05 7.040704e-05 4.041180e-05 -3.717098e-05 2.136472e-05 -8.9211
39e-05
9  -9.317359e-04 3.888107e-03 2.238822e-03 -2.047639e-03 1.181077e-03 -4.9285
99e-03
10 -2.009153e+00 7.948666e+00 4.481626e+00 -4.057354e+00           NaN
NaN
12 -8.677669e-03 3.621166e-02 2.085114e-02 -1.907057e-02 1.099989e-02 -4.5902
22e-02
13 -6.585147e-03 2.747963e-02 1.582312e-02 -1.447192e-02           NaN
NaN
14 -2.901227e-01 1.210673e+00 6.971214e-01 -6.375912e-01           NaN
NaN
15 -3.787812e-01 1.580643e+00 9.101547e-01 -8.324326e-01           NaN
NaN
17 -1.486716e-04 6.204021e-04 3.572355e-04 -3.267296e-04 1.884574e-04 -7.8642
72e-04
18 -1.166247e-03 4.866714e-03 2.802317e-03 -2.563015e-03           NaN
NaN
19 -6.372897e-03 2.658922e-02 1.530939e-02 -1.400161e-02 8.273611e-03 -3.3984
49e-02
22 -1.467087e-01 6.121711e-01 3.524872e-01 -3.223830e-01 1.876423e-01 -7.7839
03e-01
23 -1.708603e+01 2.447869e+01 3.846747e+00  9.508795e-01 1.972055e+03 -2.8252
98e+03
25 -1.565052e-07 6.530915e-07 3.760585e-07 -3.439453e-07 1.983874e-07 -8.2786
46e-07
27 -1.847225e-01 7.708414e-01 4.438604e-01 -4.059573e-01 2.341558e-01 -9.7712
54e-01
28 -6.586600e-09 2.748569e-08 1.582661e-08 -1.447511e-08           NaN
NaN
29 -5.517118e-01 7.905854e-01 1.243419e-01  3.056996e-02 6.367128e+01 -9.1219
97e+01
30 -7.887030e-12 3.291234e-11 1.895135e-11 -1.733301e-11 9.997670e-12 -4.1719
98e-11
33 -1.467087e-01 6.121711e-01 3.524872e-01 -3.223830e-01 1.876423e-01 -7.7839
03e-01
35 -2.151441e-09 8.977900e-09 5.169591e-09 -4.728137e-09 2.727186e-09 -1.1380
47e-08
36 -2.746187e-01 1.145976e+00 6.598676e-01 -6.035186e-01           NaN
```

```
NaN
             [,7]          [,8]          [,9]         [,10]         [,11]
[,12]
1             NaN           NaN -6.501269e-04  2.712960e-03  1.562158e-03 -1.4
28758e-03
3  -5.832527e+00  5.334462e+00           NaN           NaN           NaN
NaN
6             NaN           NaN -6.627367e-04  2.765581e-03  1.592457e-03 -1.4
56470e-03
7  -5.123156e-05  4.707983e-05           NaN           NaN           NaN
NaN
9  -2.837951e-03  2.595606e-03 -2.411377e-01  1.006260e+00  5.794178e-01 -5.2
99388e-01
10            NaN           NaN -4.788472e+02  1.998225e+03  1.150606e+03 -1.0
52352e+03
12 -2.643109e-02  2.417402e-02           NaN           NaN           NaN
NaN
13            NaN           NaN -1.704267e+00  7.111857e+00  4.095099e+00 -3.7
45401e+00
14            NaN           NaN -7.508513e+01  3.133280e+02  1.804183e+02 -1.6
50116e+02
15            NaN           NaN -9.803039e+01  4.090779e+02  2.355523e+02 -2.1
54375e+02
17 -4.528349e-04  4.141654e-04           NaN           NaN           NaN
NaN
18            NaN           NaN -3.018303e-01  1.259529e+00  7.252529e-01 -6.6
33204e-01
19 -1.945028e-02  1.773770e-02           NaN           NaN           NaN
NaN
22 -4.471926e-01  4.085624e-01           NaN           NaN           NaN
NaN
23 -4.439798e+02 -1.097581e+02  3.800155e-01 -5.211219e-01 -6.702756e-02 -4.0
32109e-02
25 -4.766952e-07  4.359881e-07           NaN           NaN           NaN
NaN
27 -5.626414e-01  5.145950e-01 -4.780705e+01  1.994974e+02  1.148732e+02 -1.0
50637e+02
28            NaN           NaN -1.704643e-06  7.113427e-06  4.096003e-06 -3.7
46228e-06
29 -1.433484e+01 -3.543565e+00           NaN           NaN           NaN
NaN
30 -2.402290e-11  2.197148e-11           NaN           NaN           NaN
NaN
33 -4.471926e-01  4.085624e-01           NaN           NaN           NaN
NaN
35 -6.553019e-09  5.993429e-09           NaN           NaN           NaN
NaN
36            NaN           NaN -7.107262e+01  2.965839e+02  1.707769e+02 -1.5
61935e+02


$startweights
$startweights[[1]]
$startweights[[1]][[1]]
            [,1]       [,2]       [,3]
[1,] -0.56047565  1.7150650  1.2240818
[2,] -0.23017749  0.4609162  0.3598138
[3,]  1.55870831 -1.2650612  0.4007715
[4,]  0.07050839 -0.6868529  0.1106827
[5,]  0.12928774 -0.4456620 -0.5558411

$startweights[[1]][[2]]
           [,1]       [,2]       [,3]
[1,]  1.7869131 -0.4727914 -0.7288912
[2,]  0.4978505 -1.0678237 -0.6250393
[3,] -1.9666172 -0.2179749 -1.6866933
[4,]  0.7013559 -1.0260044  0.8377870
```

```
$result.matrix
                                         [,1]
error                            5.695423e+00
reached.threshold                9.938345e-03
steps                            1.259200e+04
Intercept.to.1layhid1           -7.752387e+00
Age.to.1layhid1                 -6.802558e+01
Stage.to.1layhid1                9.745802e+01
Ki67.index.....to.1layhid1       1.531498e+01
p53.to.1layhid1                  3.786085e+00
Intercept.to.1layhid2            2.012775e+00
Age.to.1layhid2                  2.957924e+00
Stage.to.1layhid2               -1.234333e+01
Ki67.index.....to.1layhid2      -7.107448e+00
p53.to.1layhid2                  6.500512e+00
Intercept.to.1layhid3            1.431761e+02
Age.to.1layhid3                  4.364644e+01
Stage.to.1layhid3               -2.590237e+02
Ki67.index.....to.1layhid3       3.617958e+01
p53.to.1layhid3                  2.676643e+02
Intercept.to.Intermediate       -1.462353e-02
1layhid1.to.Intermediate         1.068718e+01
1layhid2.to.Intermediate        -4.871575e+00
1layhid3.to.Intermediate        -1.222856e+01
Intercept.to.Long               -2.693631e-02
1layhid1.to.Long                -1.233508e+03
1layhid2.to.Long                 6.175252e+00
1layhid3.to.Long                 1.298730e+01
Intercept.to.Short              -8.191157e+00
1layhid1.to.Short               -2.430188e-01
1layhid2.to.Short               -1.260787e+03
1layhid3.to.Short                3.852694e+01

attr(,"class")
[1] "nn"
```

This detailed output of the model shows the functions used by the model to learn from the training set and how it predicts the results for this training data. In addition, it shows which features were excluded from creating the model, and it shows the starting weights and the final optimized weights reached by the model. What is stored in the results matrix can be considered as the most important part of the model output. It shows the error of the cost function, number of steps it took the model to reach that error and learning threshold, and the final weights between the nodes. What is stored in the results matrix can be simplified in a plot:

```
> plot(NN1)
```

A look at the plot of the NN1 model (Fig. 13.2) shows the weight assigned to each neuron as an input for the next neuron. For each layer acting as an input for a next layer, there is a node in blue representing the bias, or the intercept as shown in Eq. (15.1). We can also find the steps the model took to train the data to reach the aimed threshold and the error of the cost function of the model. This error shows how well our model is being trained based on the training data set. Even though a lower error rate can be promising, it does not always translate into a higher accuracy of the model. In order to find the accuracy of the model, like previous chapters, we test the accuracy of its predictions on unseen data, which are the test data. For this purpose, we need to create

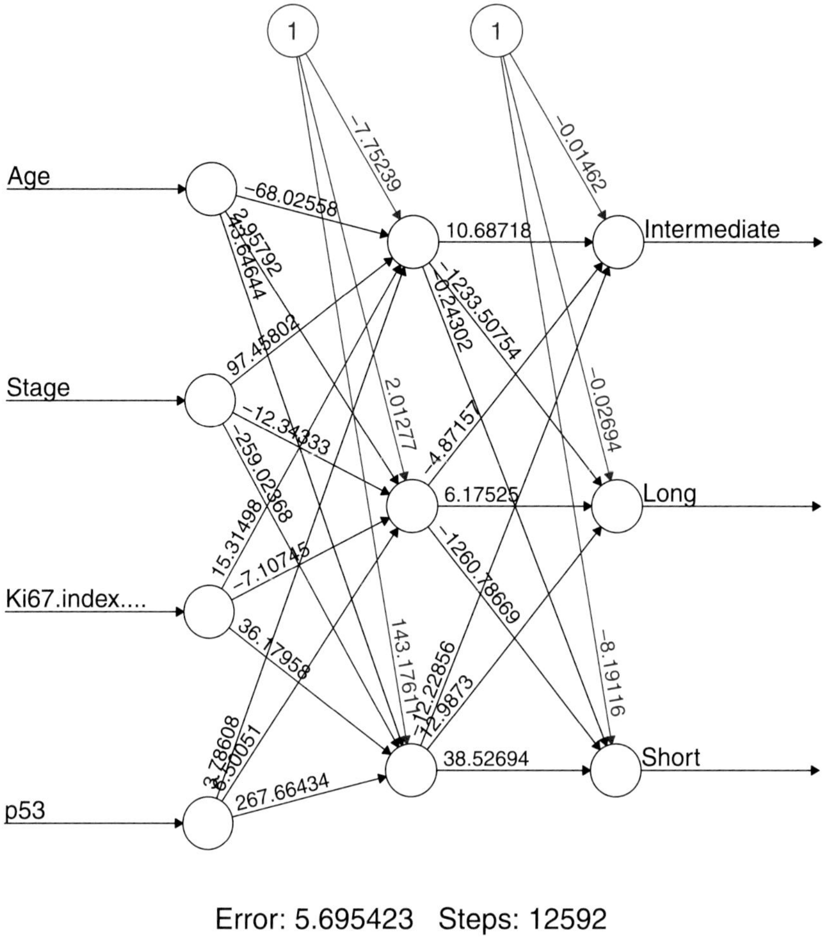

FIGURE 13.2 Plot of a neural network with one hidden layer composed of three nodes. The arrows demonstrate the assigned weights.

the confusion matrix. However, creating the confusion matrix for our neural network predictions requires a few more lines of coding compared to previous chapters. Neural networks, similar to many other classification algorithms, find the probability of an observation belonging to either of the possible categories of the dependent variable. Based on the threshold we choose for our model, these probabilities are taken into account to find to which category of the dependent variable the observation is assigned to. Like previous chapters, we use the R built-in function to make predictions using our model. We use a testing subset to evaluate how accurately our model predicts classes when faced with unseen data:

```
> Predict1=predict(NN1, test)
> Predict1
           [,1] [,2]          [,3]
2  3.691085e-08    1  0.000000e+00
4  2.034946e-02    0 3.280734e-248
5  3.722990e-08    1  0.000000e+00
8  9.999768e-01    0  2.172649e-04
11 3.691085e-08    1  0.000000e+00
16 3.691954e-08    1  0.000000e+00
20 1.742182e-01    0  1.000000e+00
21 1.292949e-07    1  0.000000e+00
24 3.691085e-08    1  0.000000e+00
26 3.691085e-08    1  0.000000e+00
31 1.735923e-01    0  1.000000e+00
32 9.999768e-01    0  1.780934e-04
34 1.742001e-01    0  1.000000e+00
34 7.632100e-01 2.867439e-01 1.931510e-03
```

As was mentioned, the model returns probabilities of the observation belonging to each of the dependent variable categories. In order to assign categories, we need to define a threshold so that the category with higher probability than the threshold will be chosen as the class of the observation. We set this threshold of probability to 0.5, and in order to convert probabilities into binary values, we use the ifelse() function as described in Chapter 4:

```
> pred1 <- ifelse(Predict1 > 0.5, 1, 0)
> pred1
   [,1] [,2] [,3]
2     0    1    0
4     0    0    0
5     0    1    0
8     1    0    0
11    0    1    0
16    0    1    0
20    0    0    1
21    0    1    0
24    0    1    0
26    0    1    0
31    0    0    1
32    1    0    0
34    0    0    1
```

If we try to build the confusion matrix at this step, we will face an error, as the class of the "pred1" output is a matrix of arrays, and its dimensions are different from the actual class of observations stored in the "Survival" column of the testing subset:

```
> class(pred1)
[1] "matrix" "array"
> dim(pred1)
[1] 13  3
```

For this reason, in order to create the confusion matrix, we change the class of the "pred1" from matrix to data frame and add a new column comparable to that of the "Survival" column of the test data. A look at the structure of the "Survival" column in our data shows that "1" is assigned to class "Intermediate," "2" is assigned to "Long," and "3" is assigned to "Short." In order to make the "pred1" output comparable to the test data, we need to ensure that this structure is conserved in the "pred1" output, so comparisons will not be misleading. Therefore, we create a column in "pred1" called "Survival," and when [, 1] is 1 and for observations, we label it "Intermediate," and so forth.

```
> pred1 <- as.data.frame(pred1)
> pred1$Survival[pred1$V1==1]="Intermediate"
> pred1$Survival[pred1$V2==1]="Long"
> pred1$Survival[pred1$V3==1]="Short"
> pred1$Survival <- as.factor(pred1$Survival)
```

Now we can use the confusionMatrix() function from the "caret" package [15]:

```
> library(caret)
> confusionMatrix(pred1$Survival,test$Survival)
Confusion Matrix and Statistics

              Reference
Prediction     Intermediate Long Short
  Intermediate            2    0     0
  Long                    0    6     1
  Short                   1    1     1

Overall Statistics

               Accuracy : 0.75
                 95% CI : (0.4281, 0.9451)
    No Information Rate : 0.5833
    P-Value [Acc > NIR] : 0.1916

                  Kappa : 0.5663

 Mcnemar's Test P-Value : NA

Statistics by Class:

                     Class: Intermediate Class: Long Class: Short
Sensitivity                       0.6667      0.8571      0.50000
Specificity                       1.0000      0.8000      0.80000
Pos Pred Value                    1.0000      0.8571      0.33333
Neg Pred Value                    0.9000      0.8000      0.88889
Prevalence                        0.2500      0.5833      0.16667
Detection Rate                    0.1667      0.5000      0.08333
Detection Prevalence              0.1667      0.5833      0.25000
Balanced Accuracy                 0.8333      0.8286      0.65000
```

A comparison of the results from our neural network predictive model with other classification models reveals that a neural network does not perform significantly better than previous models, and in some cases, its performance might be slightly poorer than other models. One of the reasons for this is the small size of the training and testing data sets. As mentioned earlier, neural networks are able to handle large dimensional data sets and capture several aspects of the relationships between the covariates and the dependent variable. However, it may be better to reserve their use for such data sets, rather than smaller data sets, which can be easily handled with other machine learning algorithms. Use of neural networks, in addition to not yielding better results, is more demanding in terms of the time elapsed to train the model and computational cost and memory. In addition to the fact that neural networks require more time and memory compared to other algorithms, the structure of a neural network in terms of complexity, which is determined by the number of hidden layers and number of neurons in each layer, affects the computational costs of creating the neural networks. These costs need to be weighed against the improvement in the performance of the model when making the decision on its complexity. In order to see if the complexity of a model can improve its performance, we create a second neural network, NN2, which is similar to our NN1 model, except for the number of its hidden layers. We use the same parameters to create the model and fix the effects of randomization. Furthermore, the same training and testing data will be used to train and test the model.

```
set.seed(123)
NN2 <- neuralnet(Survival~., data=train,
                        hidden=c(4,2,4), act.fct = "logistic",
                        linear.output = F, err.fct="ce", threshold = 0.01)
```

In order to compare learning of the two models from the training data, we call the error of cost function, the threshold of the error to be reached by the model, and the steps taken to train the model. We can overlook the rest of the details from the model output as a comparison of the weights assigned to nodes is critical to compare our models with different layers. So we only call the first three objects from the results matrix, which represent error of the cost function, threshold, and number of steps taken for training the model, respectively:

```
> NN2$result.matrix[c(1:3),]
           error reached.threshold            steps
    5.783494e+00        9.567163e-03     1.570000e+02
```

A comparison of the error from the cost function of the two models shows that convoluting the model did not enhance the model's learning from the training data. However, making a decision on the performance of the model merely based on its error rate is not possible. In order to further investigate whether increasing the model's convolution level will be cost-effective in terms of performance and accuracy, we compare the accuracy of NN2 and NN1.

```
> Predict2=predict(NN2, test)
> pred2 <- ifelse(Predict2 > 0.5, 1, 0)
> pred2 <- as.data.frame(pred2)
> pred2$Survival[pred2$V1==1]="Intermediate"
> pred2$Survival[pred2$V2==1]="Long"
> pred2$Survival[pred2$V3==1]="Short"
> pred2$Survival <- as.factor(pred2$Survival)
> confusionMatrix(pred2$Survival,test$Survival)
Confusion Matrix and Statistics

              Reference
Prediction     Intermediate Long Short
  Intermediate            0    0     0
  Long                    1    6     0
  Short                   2    2     2

Overall Statistics

               Accuracy : 0.6154
                 95% CI : (0.3158, 0.8614)
    No Information Rate : 0.6154
    P-Value [Acc > NIR] : 0.6194

                  Kappa : 0.3564

 Mcnemar's Test P-Value : 0.1718

Statistics by Class:

                     Class: Intermediate Class: Long Class: Short
Sensitivity                       0.0000      0.7500       1.0000
Specificity                       1.0000      0.8000       0.6364
Pos Pred Value                       NaN      0.8571       0.3333
Neg Pred Value                    0.7692      0.6667       1.0000
Prevalence                        0.2308      0.6154       0.1538
Detection Rate                    0.0000      0.4615       0.1538
Detection Prevalence              0.0000      0.5385       0.4615
Balanced Accuracy
```

The accuracy of the model is not improved compared to the accuracy of NN1. This makes the decision regarding the complexity of the model easy in this case, as more complexity did not result in improvement of the model's performance. Even for instances where the accuracy of the model is increased with increased complexity of the model, this increase of accuracy must be weighed against the computational requirements of creating more complex data. This can be particularly true for high-dimensional data sets as the time and computation costs will increase dramatically; however, in larger data sets, it is more probable for the model to improve in accuracy if the level of complexity is increased. As both training and testing data sets are both small, the predictions cannot reflect how good the model can be. A similar model trained on larger training and testing data sets with a balanced proportion of classes will yield better results as effects of each misclassification will be smaller on the final results. Furthermore, the model will have more examples to be trained upon.

Considering these limitations in the training and testing data, let us make an attempt to improve the results by changing parameters of the model. We will create a third neural network classification model, NN3, using backpropagation. Backpropagation, as mentioned earlier, is one of the strongest and most common methods for improving model performance. In this method, the contribution of each node to the cost function is calculated, and the weights assigned to nodes with higher error rates will be lowered to mitigate their effects in the final results of the model. This method is specifically appropriate for complex neural networks with multiple hidden layers. In order to compare the results of a model tuned with backpropagation with that of a feedforward neural network, we maintain the rest of the arguments and parameters of training the model similar to NN2.

```
> set.seed(123)
> NN3 <- neuralnet(Survival~., data=train,
+                    hidden=c(4, 2, 4), act.fct = "logistic", algorithm
= "backprop",
+                    learningrate= 0.02, linear.output = F,
err.fct="ce", threshold = 0.01)
```

When tuning models with backpropagation, the learning rate of the model needs to be specified. Learning rate determines the rate of changes in the model when better weights are assigned to the nodes in the model. In order to compare the errors from backpropagation with errors from the feedforward model, we call the error rate of the NN3:

```
> NN3$result.matrix[1,]
     error
0.07564467
```

In this case, the model's error has been decreased. Even though this is a promising factor, we still need to compare the accuracy of the results using the test data.

```
> Predict3=predict(NN3, test)
> pred3 <- ifelse(Predict3 > 0.5, 1, 0)
> pred3 <- as.data.frame(pred3)
> pred3$Survival[pred3$V1==1]="Intermediate"
> pred3$Survival[pred3$V2==1]="Long"
> pred3$Survival[pred3$V3==1]="Short"
> pred3$Survival <- as.factor(pred3$Survival)
> confusionMatrix(pred3$Survival,test$Survival)
Confusion Matrix and Statistics

              Reference
Prediction     Intermediate Long Short
  Intermediate            0    2     0
  Long                    1    6     1
  Short                   2    0     1

Overall Statistics

               Accuracy : 0.5385
                 95% CI : (0.2513, 0.8078)
    No Information Rate : 0.6154
    P-Value [Acc > NIR] : 0.8051

                  Kappa : 0.1613

 Mcnemar's Test P-Value : 0.3430

Statistics by Class:

                     Class: Intermediate Class: Long Class: Short
Sensitivity                       0.0000      0.7500      0.50000
Specificity                       0.8000      0.6000      0.81818
Pos Pred Value                    0.0000      0.7500      0.33333
Neg Pred Value                    0.7273      0.6000      0.90000
Prevalence                        0.2308      0.6154      0.15385
Detection Rate                    0.0000      0.4615      0.07692
Detection Prevalence              0.1538      0.6154      0.23077
Balanced Accuracy                 0.4000      0.6750      0.65909
```

The accuracy of the model is not increased. Even though these observations are helpful with making a decision regarding the structure of the neural network, or whether choosing a neural network for making predictions in the first place, we must remember that similar changes in the results may not be observed for different data sets. For our data, given the size of the data set, and the relationship of variables with one another, neural networks did not provide better results compared to other algorithms such as linear regression or random forests. However, neural networks are still among the most useful methods for handling large data sets. More examples in Chapter 14 will allow a better comparison of the machine learning models and neural networks.

In the models created thus far, the stage of the disease was not treated as a categorical variable since neural networks do not take as input categorical variables. Therefore we need to change the categorical variables in a way that can be taken by the neural networks. As mentioned earlier, one of the most common methods of handling categorical variables when making neural network models is one-hot encoding. In order to get familiar with this method, we treat the stage of the disease as a categorical variable similar to previous chapters.

There are several methods and packages for one-hot encoding. We use the dummyVars() function of the "caret" package for this purpose. For this purpose, we need to change the "Stage" variable into a categorical variable. One-hot encoding renders any categorical variable in a data set to a binary variable; therefore we need to exclude the dependent variable, which is also a categorical variable, before our one-hot encoding, and then recreate the entire data set after one-hot encoding of the stage variable. In order to recreate our entire data set after one-hot encoding, we create a data frame of the column representing the dependent variable, to merge this data frame with the data frame of the one-hot encoded variables using the cbind() function:

```
> str(data)
'data.frame':   36 obs. of  5 variables:
 $ Age              : int  42 2 34 6 32 15 65 23 63 13 ...
 $ Stage            : int  3 1 2 2 2 4 2 4 3 2 ...
 $ Ki67.index....: int  78 12 46 63 83 80 15 78 51 46 ...
 $ p53              : int  6 0 2 11 23 28 1 13 0 1 ...
 $ Survival         : chr  "Intermediate" "Long" "Long" "Long" ...
> Survival <- data.frame(data$Survival)
> data <-data[,-5]
> data$Stage <- as.factor(data$Stage)
```

Now our data set is ready to be transformed using one-hot encoding using the "caret" package:

```
> library(caret)
> dummy <- dummyVars(" ~ .", data=data)
> newdata <- data.frame(predict(dummy, newdata = data))
> head(newdata)
  Age Stage.1 Stage.2 Stage.3 Stage.4 Ki67.index.... p53
1  42       0       0       1       0             78   6
2   2       1       0       0       0             12   0
3  34       0       1       0       0             46   2
4   6       0       1       0       0             63  11
5  32       0       1       0       0             83  23
6  15       0       0       0       1             80  28
```

Now we merge the "Survival" data frame with "newdata," and transform the class of the new column into categorical:

```
> data <- cbind(newdata, Survival)
> colnames(data)[8] <- "Survival"
> data$Survival <- as.factor(data$Survival)
```

Similar to other neural networks, we need to standardize the data set by selecting numeric columns:

```
> data[,c(1, 6, 7)] <- scale(data[,c(1, 6, 7)], scale= T, center= T)
```

Now our data set is ready to be divided into training and testing subsets:

```
> set.seed(123)
> subsets <- sample(2, nrow(data), prob=c(0.7, 0.3), replace=T)
> train <- data[subsets==1,]
> test <- data[subsets==2,]
> NN_OHE <- neuralnet(Survival~., data=train,
+                            hidden=3, act.fct = "logistic",
+                            linear.output = F)
```

In order to compare the performance of our model with that of NN1, we call the error and accuracy of NN_OHE:

```
> NN_OHE$result.matrix[1,]
    error
0.5489979
> Predict_OHE=predict(NN_OHE, test)
> pred_OHE <- ifelse(Predict_OHE > 0.5, 1, 0)
> pred_OHE <- as.data.frame(pred_OHE)
> pred_OHE$Survival[pred_OHE$V1==1]="Intermediate"
> pred_OHE$Survival[pred_OHE$V2==1]="Long"
> pred_OHE$Survival[pred_OHE$V3==1]="Short"
> pred_OHE$Survival <- as.factor(pred_OHE$Survival)
> confusionMatrix(pred_OHE$Survival,test$Survival)
Confusion Matrix and Statistics

              Reference
Prediction     Intermediate Long Short
  Intermediate            2    1     0
  Long                    0    6     0
  Short                   1    1     2

Overall Statistics

               Accuracy : 0.7692
                 95% CI : (0.4619, 0.9496)
    No Information Rate : 0.6154
    P-Value [Acc > NIR] : 0.1986

                  Kappa : 0.625

 Mcnemar's Test P-Value : 0.3916

Statistics by Class:

                     Class: Intermediate Class: Long Class: Short
Sensitivity                       0.6667      0.7500       1.0000
Specificity                       0.9000      1.0000       0.8182
Pos Pred Value                    0.6667      1.0000       0.5000
Neg Pred Value                    0.9000      0.7143       1.0000
Prevalence                        0.2308      0.6154       0.1538
Detection Rate                    0.1538      0.4615       0.1538
Detection Prevalence              0.2308      0.4615       0.3077
Balanced  Accuracy                0.7833      0.8750       0.9091
```

The error rate of NN-OHE is smaller than that of NN1, and their accuracies are comparable at 75% versus 76%. This reflects that one-hot encoding of categorical variables can result in better performance of the models in general. However, in our case, as our categorical variable was in nature denoted by an ordinal number, which inversely affects the survival outcome, the accuracies of the two models are comparable. It must be noted that for data sets with categorical independent variables, one-hot encoding or using other methods of transforming categorical variables for use by neural networks is necessary.

Neural networks for regression problems

In previous sections of this chapter, different methods for developing neural network classifiers were overviewed, and their performance was compared with one another and other classifiers developed in previous chapters. We now overview neural networks for regression problems using the same data set as used for regression throughout this book. We then compare the performance of neural networks with other regression models.

We start off by preparing our data set to create training and testing subsets. A recall on the structure of the data set shows that the "Stage" of the disease must be treated as a categorical variable.

```
> reg_data$Stage <- as.factor(reg_data$Stage)
> str(reg_data)
'data.frame':   36 obs. of  5 variables:
 $ Age          : int  42 2 34 6 32 15 65 23 63 13 ...
 $ Stage        : Factor w/ 4 levels "1","2","3","4": 3 1 2 2 2 4 2 4 3 2 ..
.
 $ Ki67.index....: int  78 12 46 63 83 80 15 78 51 46 ...
 $ p53          : int  6 0 2 11 23 28 1 13 0 1 ...
 $ Survival     : int  13 102 43 12 5 1 45 7 41 23 ...
```

Now we need to transform the "Stage" variable into binary variables so it can be taken as input by neural networks.

```
> dummy <- dummyVars(" ~ .", data=reg_data)
> reg_newdata <- data.frame(predict(dummy, newdata = reg_data))
> str(reg_newdata)
'data.frame':   36 obs. of  8 variables:
 $ Age          : num  42 2 34 6 32 15 65 23 63 13 ...
 $ Stage.1      : num  0 1 0 0 0 0 0 0 0 0 ...
 $ Stage.2      : num  0 0 1 1 1 0 1 0 0 1 ...
 $ Stage.3      : num  1 0 0 0 0 0 0 0 1 0 ...
 $ Stage.4      : num  0 0 0 0 0 1 0 1 0 0 ...
 $ Ki67.index....: num  78 12 46 63 83 80 15 78 51 46 ...
 $ p53          : num  6 0 2 11 23 28 1 13 0 1 ...
 $ Survival     : num  13 102 43 12 5 1 45 7 41 23 ...
```

Before dividing our data set into training and testing subsets, we need to standardize numeric variables:

```
> reg_newdata[,c(1, 6, 7)] <- scale(reg_newdata[,c(1, 6, 7)], scale= T, cente
r= T)
> set.seed(123)
> subsets <- sample(2, nrow(reg_newdata), prob=c(0.7, 0.3), replace=T)
> reg_train <- reg_newdata[subsets==1,]
> reg_test <- reg_newdata[subsets==2,]
```

Now we can train our neural networks using the training subset and test its performance when faced with unseen data using our testing subset:

```
> reg_NN <- neuralnet(Survival~., data=reg_train,
+                     hidden=3, act.fct = "logistic",
+                     linear.output = F)
```

Now we need to understand different parameters about our model. Important parameters of our model include the error rate, and, similar to other regression models, we will call our model's root mean square error (RMSE). Even though we cannot compare the error rate of neural networks with other regression models developed in previous chapters, we can compare the RMSE of neural networks with other regression models, which is one of the most important aspects of comparing different regression models.

```
> reg_NN$result.matrix[1,]
   error
19433.51
```

A look at the error rate of the neural networks shows a relatively large error rate, giving us an idea of how well the neural networks can learn based on the training data. However, the model's RMSE when predicting observations in the testing subset is a better judge of its performance. In order to calculate the RMSE, we use the rmse() function from the "Metrics" package [16]:

```
> library(Metrics)
> reg_predict <- predict(reg_NN, reg_test)
> RMSE_NN <- rmse(reg_predict, reg_test$Survival)
> RMSE_NN
[1] 41.95695
```

RMSE for our model is higher compared to models trained using other algorithms. One of the reasons for this observation is that our data can be linearly separable, which is why it is better predicted by methods such as linear regression. The other reason is the structure of the data set. Neural networks demonstrate their best performance when reserved for high-dimensional data sets.

Unsupervised neural networks

Every algorithm discussed thus far was among the supervised learning algorithms where labeled data are used to train a model, which can be used for the prediction of unseen data with similar features in the future. Machine learning and neural network algorithms can help us beyond making predictions, by helping us understand the relationships among different components of the data sets. Unsupervised learning helps us with understanding these relationships, which have several applications when working with large data sets, which have been overviewed in Chapter 5.

In this chapter, we briefly overview one of the unsupervised neural network algorithms, SOMs, also known as Kohonen maps. These algorithms are particularly useful for dimensionality reduction, and they are extensively used for better understanding and representation of biological data sets, such as microarray data, next-generation sequencing, and flow cytometry, to name a few [17]. However, it must be noted that the term dimensionality reduction used here is different from dimensionality reduction in that here it is a method of data aggregation rather than choosing features for deconvolution of data. Unlike neural networks that have hidden layers, SOMs have only input layer and output layer. The input layer, similar to neural networks, can have as many nodes as data features. However, the output layer is always a two-dimensional lattice or map of neurons that represent the input data [17]. In this map, data points are categorized into different homogeneous groups based on their similar features. This results in the presentation of high-dimensional large data sets in a two-dimensional map, which will be much easier to interpret and help with understanding the relationships between features and data sets.

As mentioned earlier, each input layer of the SOMs represents one of the variables in the data sets. Each neuron in the two-dimensional output layer receives a weight for each data point for every feature, as depicted in Fig. 13.3. Unlike supervised neural network models, however, the output layers do not require an activation function to represent the weights. The weights corresponding to each feature from each data point are not summed up to be represented by an output neuron. Rather, these weights are considered as coordinates of the output neuron. For each data point, the neuron in the output layer that is closest to the data point is found using different distance measuring functions such as a Euclidean function. This output neuron is called the best-matching unit (BMU). Once the BMU is found, in order to decrease the distance between the BMU and the data point, weights assigned to the data point are adjusted. The adjustment of weights for each data point depends on the distance between the data point and the BMU—the smaller this distance is, the more significant the adjustment of weights will be. As there are several BMUs for each data set, data

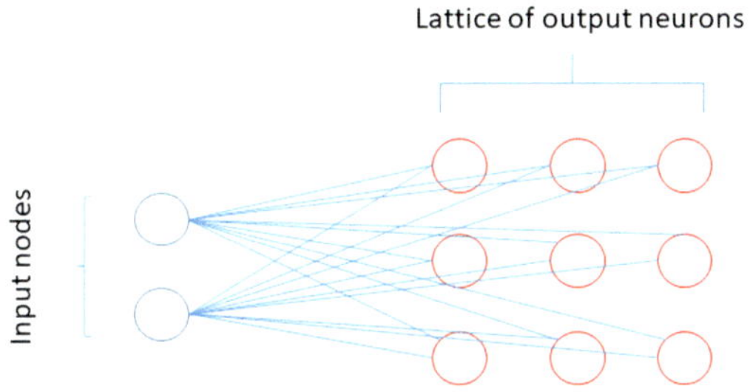

FIGURE 13.3 Schematic of self-organizing maps (SOMs). Any number of input features can be represented in a two-dimensional map of neurons.

points can be affected by several BMUs, and the magnitude of these effects is determined by how close each BMU is to a data point. As this process goes on, the specified radius in which data point weights are adjusted will decrease for each BMU. Therefore each BMU will have its own territory composed of data points sharing the same feature, and they will be represented similarly in the two-dimensional map. This leads to a better representation of relationships in the data set, which would be hard to interpret otherwise [17].

Even though SOMs are appreciated more when used for representing large data sets when they reach their full potential, for demonstrative purposes, we used the same data set that was used for training supervised classification models. However, as SOMs are unsupervised learning algorithms, we need to exclude the labels of each data point before training the model:

```
> str(data)
'data.frame':   36 obs. of  5 variables:
 $ Age           : int  42 2 34 6 32 15 65 23 63 13 ...
 $ Stage         : int  3 1 2 2 2 4 2 4 3 2 ...
 $ Ki67.index....: int  78 12 46 63 83 80 15 78 51 46 ...
 $ p53           : int  6 0 2 11 23 28 1 13 0 1 ...
 $ Survival      : chr  "Intermediate" "Long" "Long" "Long" ...
> data <- data[,-5]
```

Similar to supervised neural networks, we need to scale our data set in order to prevent biases in assigned weights due to different variable units and scales. Similar to neural networks, SOMs cannot handle categorical variables unless they are converted into binary variables using methods such as one-hot encoding. However, some variants of SOMs, such as Frequency Neuron Mixed Self-Organizing Map [18], can deal with both numeric and categorical variables, which are beyond the scope of this chapter. Similar to the case for supervised neural networks, as our categorical variable is represented by numbers in nature, we can opt to either render our categorical variable by one-hot encoding or treat it as a numeric variable; we opt for the latter in this chapter. In order to employ SOMs for our data set, we use one of the most common and simple R packages for SOMs, the "kohonen" package [19].

```
> install.packages("kohonen")
> library(kohonen)
```

Similar to other neural networks, we need to fix the effect of randomization using the set.seed() function. In order to create an SOM, we will need to define grid units, which will be used for demonstrating the SOMs. This grid is defined by the somgrid() function of the "kohonen" package. We will then need to set up the neural network parameters for learning of the SOM. Before developing our SOM, we need to ensure that the "Rccp" package is updated.

```
> set.seed(123)
> som_grid <- somgrid(xdim=3, ydim=3, topo="rectangular")
> SOMap <- som(scaled, grid= som_grid, alpha= c(0.05, 0.01),
+              radius= 2)
```

In this function, we need to define the data and the grid that will be used for training the data set. We need to determine the learning rate of the algorithm, which denotes the amount of changes in the weights after several iterations, which infinitely will approach zero. The default value for learning rate, which is determined by alpha, is 0.05 and 0.01, which means that after several iterations, this value will decrease from 0.05 to 0.01. Radius can be determined by the analyst, which determines the distance from BMU for affecting neighboring data sets. Throughout the learning process, radius will change linearly to zero, as throughout learning adjustment of weights brings BMUs and data points together.

Plotting SOMs is an important aspect of implementing them. There are several ways to plot SOMs, and we will overview some of them.

```
plot(SOMap, type="changes")
```

This plot (Fig. 13.4) shows that the mean distance between BMUs and data points is gradually decreasing from 0.11 to 0.07 over 100 iterations.

The main plots in SOMs are the ones that allow a two-dimensional map of the data set. There are several methods to make such plots, and in this chapter, we overview only a few of them. We start off by the easiest plot in terms of programming, known as the Codes plot, which provides useful information regarding the relationship of features with one another (Fig. 13.5).

```
> plot(SOMap)
```

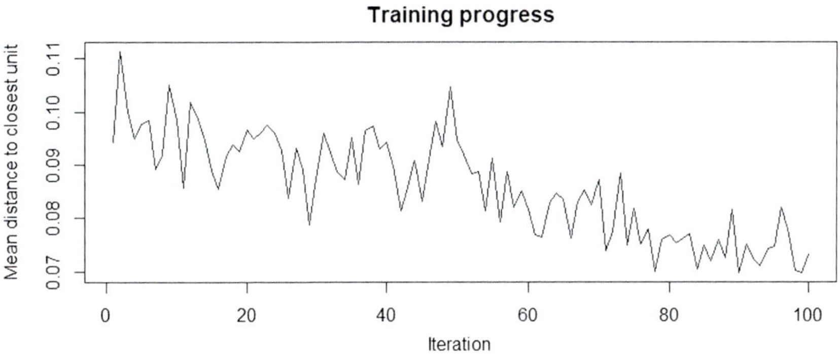

FIGURE 13.4 Plot of changes in mean distance to closest best-matching unit. Over several number of iterations, this distance decreases.

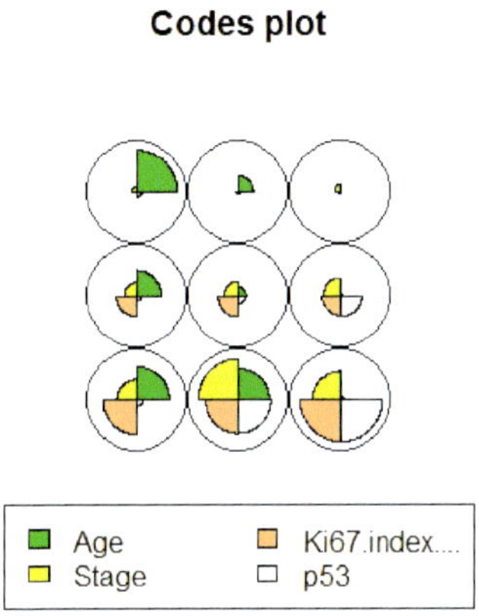

FIGURE 13.5 Codes plot demonstrating the importance of each feature for each group divided based on similarity of features.

This plot is a lattice of nine neurons, each representing a group of data points with similar features. In the first node, for example, age and Ki67 index of patients are similarly high in these group of patients, while these patients are of lower stages and p53 expression is quite low in them. This lattice of neurons shows us how our patients can be divided into nine groups in a way that they represent similar characteristics.

We can also observe how many data points each of these neurons represents. Various plots can demonstrate such information (Figs. 13.6 and 13.7).

```
> plot(SOMap, type= "mapping")
> plot(SOMap, type= "count")
```

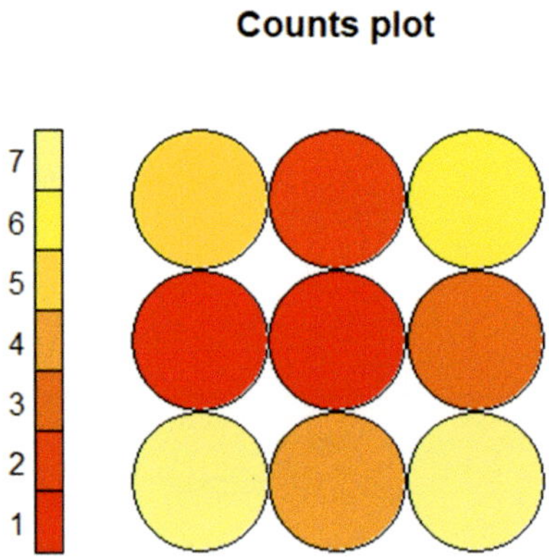

FIGURE 13.6 Counts plot demonstrating color coded number of observations in each neuron.

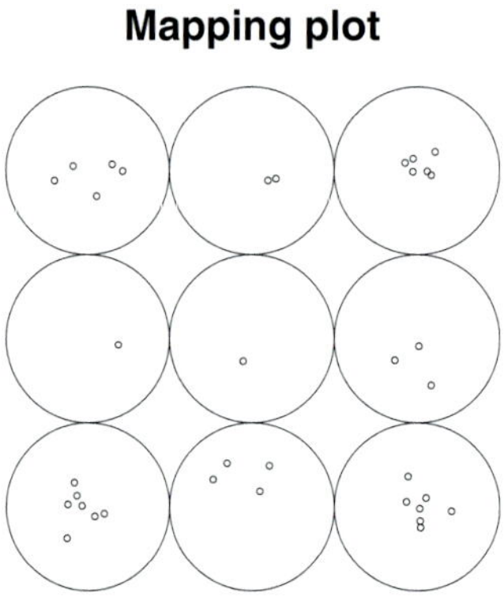

FIGURE 13.7 Mapping plot demonstrating the number of observations in each of the neurons.

The first plot shows the number of data points represented by each neuron, and the second plot color codes these numbers. A combination of SOM plots can help discover new patterns in data, which can be used in the concept of biological data, which have several applications, including diagnosis, discovery of new therapeutic targets, and classification of diseases, among several others [20].

References

[1] R.Y. Choi, A.S. Coyner, J. Kalpathy-Cramer, M.F. Chiang, J.P. Campbell, Introduction to machine learning, neural networks, and deep learning, Translational Vision Science & Technology 9 (2) (2020) 14. Available from: https://doi.org/10.1167/tvst.9.2.14.

[2] M. Nadif, F. Role, Unsupervised and self-supervised deep learning approaches for biomedical text mining, Briefings in Bioinformatics 22 (2) (2021) 1592–1603. Available from: https://doi.org/10.1093/bib/bbab016.
[3] N. Shahid, T. Rappon, W. Berta, Applications of artificial neural networks in health care organizational decision-making: a scoping review, PLoS One 14 (2) (2019) e0212356. Available from: https://doi.org/10.1371/journal.pone.0212356.
[4] S.J. Yang, S.L. Lipnick, N.R. Makhortova, S. Venugopalan, M. Fan, Z. Armstrong, et al., Applying deep neural network analysis to high-content image-based assays, SLAS Discovery: Advancing Life Sciences R & D 24 (8) (2019) 829–841.
[5] V.C. Pezoulas, O. Hazapis, N. Lagopati, T.P. Exarchos, A.V. Goules, A.G. Tzioufas, et al., Machine learning approaches on high throughput NGS data to unveil mechanisms of function in biology and disease, Cancer Genomics & Proteomics 18 (5) (2021) 605–626. Available from: https://doi.org/10.21873/cgp.20284.
[6] H.B. Burke, Artificial neural networks for cancer research: outcome prediction, Seminars in Surgical Oncology 10 (1) (1994) 73–79. Available from: https://doi.org/10.1002/ssu.298010011.
[7] M. Mostavi, Y.C. Chiu, Y. Huang, Y. Chen, Convolutional neural network models for cancer type prediction based on gene expression, BMC Medical Genomics 13 (Suppl 5) (2020) 44. Available from: https://doi.org/10.1186/s12920-020-0677-2.
[8] S.H. Han, K.W. Kim, S. Kim, Y.C. Youn, Artificial neural network: understanding the basic concepts without mathematics, Dementia and Neurocognitive Disorders 17 (3) (2018) 83–89. Available from: https://doi.org/10.12779/dnd.2018.17.3.83.
[9] P.M. Sathe, J. Venitz, Comparison of neural network and multiple linear regression as dissolution predictors, Drug Development and Industrial Pharmacy 29 (3) (2003) 349–355. Available from: https://doi.org/10.1081/ddc-120018209.
[10] D.J. Sargent, Comparison of artificial neural networks with other statistical approaches: results from medical data sets, Cancer 91 (8 Suppl) (2001) 1636–1642. https://doi.org/10.1002/1097-0142(20010415)91:8 + <1636::aid-cncr1176>3.0.co;2-d.
[11] Vargas, V.M., Gutierrez, P.A., Barbero-Gomez, J., & Hervas-Martinez, C. (2021). Activation Functions for Convolutional Neural Networks: Proposals and Experimental Study. *IEEE transactions on neural networks and learning systems, PP*, 10.1109/TNNLS.2021.3105444. Advance online publication. Available from: https://doi.org/10.1109/TNNLS.2021.3105444.
[12] B.M. Ozyildirim, M. Avci, Logarithmic learning for generalized classifier neural network, Neural Networks: The Official Journal of the International Neural Network Society 60 (2014) 133–140. Available from: https://doi.org/10.1016/j.neunet.2014.08.004.
[13] R.J. Erb, Introduction to backpropagation neural network computation, Pharmaceutical Research 10 (2) (1993) 165–170. Available from: https://doi.org/10.1023/a:101896622.
[14] Fritsch, S., Guenther, F.,Wright, M.N., Suling, M., Mueller, S.M. (2019). neuralnet: Training of Neural Networks.
[15] M. Kuhn, Caret package, Journal of Statistical Software 28 (5) (2008).
[16] P. Schneider, Y. Tanrikulu, G. Schneider, Self-organizing maps in drug discovery: compound library design, scaffold-hopping, repurposing, Current Medicinal Chemistry 16 (3) (2009) 258–266. Available from: https://doi.org/10.2174/092986709787002655.
[17] T. Kohonen, Essentials of the self-organizing map, Neural Networks: The Official Journal of the International Neural Network Society 37 (2013) 52–65. Available from: https://doi.org/10.1016/j.neunet.2012.09.018.
[18] C.D. Coso, D. Fustes, C. Dafonte, F.J. Nóvoa, J.M. Rodríguez-Pedreira, B. Arcay, Mixing numerical and categorical data in a self-organizing map by means of frequency neurons, Applied Soft Computing 36 (2015) 246–254.

[19] R. Wehrens, J. Kruisselbrink, Flexible self-organizing maps in kohonen 3.0, Journal of Statistical Software 87 (7) (2018) 1–18. Available from: https://doi.org/10.18637/jss.v087.i07.

[20] E.M. Borkowska, A. Kruk, A. Jedrzejczyk, M. Rozniecki, Z. Jablonowski, M. Traczyk, et al., Molecular subtyping of bladder cancer using Kohonen self-organizing maps, Cancer medicine 3 (5) (2014) 1225–1234. Available from: https://doi.org/10.1002/cam4.217.

CHAPTER

14

Practice examples

Practice examples for machine learning algorithms

In previous chapters of this book, we learned the basics of some of the machine learning algorithms and briefly introduced convolutional neural networks. Similar training data made comparison of results feasible for the introduced algorithms. In this chapter, we will employ our knowledge from the previous chapters on real-world data obtained from one of the public databases introduced in Chapter 3. We aim to find genes that can predict glioblastoma patients' survival using gene expression profiles of these patients.

The data sets used in this chapter are array-based gene expression profiles of glioblastoma patients: GSE53733 and GSE83300 available on Gene Expression Omnibus (GEO). GSE53733 provides array-based expression profiles of primary glioblastoma tumors from 70 patients. These patients were divided based on their overall survival into long- ($>$36 months), intermediate- ($>$12 and $<$36 months), and short-term ($<$12 months) survivors. GSE83300 provides expression profiles of primary glioblastoma tumors from 50 patients. Survival of patients is reported in overall survival in months. A matrix of gene expressions for each of the series can be found on the corresponding webpage through "Series Matrix File(s)"; however, these matrices require some filtering in order to obtain clear expression profiles. Further information regarding each patient can be obtained through "Samples" designated by identifiers starting with "GSM" (e.g., GSM1299519).

In this chapter, we use GSE83300 to train our regression model. Performance of the regression models will be assessed through the testing subset of GSE83300. We will use GSE53733 to train and test our classification models. For both regression and classification models, in order to find significant genes, we use the "GEO2R" tool of the GEO database, which serves to identify differentially expressed genes (DEGs). Conventionally, DEGs are determined based on adjusted p values (also known as false discovery rate or FDR) and logarithm to base 2 of fold change, which is simply denoted by log FC in literature.

Immunoinformatics of Cancers
DOI: https://doi.org/10.1016/B978-0-12-822400-7.00002-6

Cutoff values of significance for log FC and FDR vary from one study to another; however, a log FC > 1 and FDR < 0.05 or 0.1 demonstrates different expressions in different studies.

Even though GEO provides a comprehensive guide on how to use GEO2R, a few points need to be remarked in this chapter. In order for GEO2R to report log FC, only two groups should be defined for comparison; therefore we compare gene expressions of patients with long survival and short survival in GSE53733, and use the same temporal criteria for comparison of GSE83300. In order to find DEGs with GEO2R, it is important for the comparison groups to be truly different in their nature; otherwise, significance thresholds for log FC and FDR will not be met.

In this chapter, as we aim to find genes associated with patient survival, we use GEO2R to find probes corresponding to genes. As both comparison groups are from glioblastoma patients, GEO2R will not return results that pass the criteria of different expressions. Therefore we consider the highest log FC as the criterion to find genes that can predict survival of glioblastoma patients.

Classification models

We start off by making our classification models. We need to first curate our data set to include both the expression profile of patients and their survival. We can make a data frame of patients' survival and use the R built-in function to merge expression profiles with the patients' survival, which will be our dependent variable.

The curated data set, which we will refer to as "expressions70" for GSE53733, will have 71 columns and 54675 rows:

```
> dim(expressions70)
[1] 54675    71
```

In order to find significant genes, we need to find the highest log FC values from the GEO2R results table:

```
> head(GEO2R)
           ID adj.P.Val  P.Value     t     B  logFC Gene.symbol
1   209511_at     0.432 1.16e-05 -5.01 1.576 -0.389      POLR2F
2   231018_at     0.432 2.04e-05  4.83 1.222  0.571       PALM3
3   204927_at     0.432 3.13e-05  4.69 0.951  0.318      RASSF7
4   229146_at     0.432 3.16e-05  4.69 0.944  0.672     C7orf31
5 215342_s_at     0.567 5.59e-05 -4.51 0.583 -0.386    RABGAP1L
6   229912_at     0.567 6.22e-05  4.47 0.514  0.613        SDK1
```

```
                              Gene.title
1            RNA polymerase II subunit F
2                           paralemmin 3
3 Ras association domain family member 7
4     chromosome 7 open reading frame 31
5    RAB GTPase activating protein 1 like
6      sidekick cell adhesion molecule 1
```

We create a new column in this data set, "abs," to represent the absolute values of log FC:

```
> GEO2R$abs <- abs(GEO2R$logFC)
```

Now we need to sort "GEO2R" based on the values of the "abs" column to find the probes with the highest absolute log FC.

```
> top <- GEO2R[order(GEO2R$abs, decreasing=T),]
> head(top)
            ID adj.P.Val   P.Value    t      B logFC Gene.symbol                    Gene.title
34  211564_s_at     0.613 0.0004914 3.79 -0.819 1.060      PDLIM4            PDZ and LIM domain 4
67    205453_at     0.613 0.0009294 3.58 -1.234 0.997       HOXB2                   homeobox B2
305 210135_s_at     0.634 0.0036540 3.09 -2.129 0.996       SHOX2       short stature homeobox 2
492 206201_s_at     0.634 0.0057537 2.92 -2.425 0.991       MEOX2          mesenchyme homeobox 2
611   226237_at     0.650 0.0072759 2.83 -2.578 0.990      COL8A1 collagen type VIII alpha 1 chain
133   203184_at     0.613 0.0015133 3.41 -1.552 0.984        FBN2                    fibrillin 2
      abs
34  1.060
67  0.997
305 0.996
492 0.991
611 0.990
133 0.984
```

Considering the number of observations in our data set, 10 features is approximately appropriate to allow discovery of important genes, yet not oversaturating our model.

```
> top10 <- top[c(1:10),]
> top10
             ID adj.P.Val    P.Value    t      B logFC Gene.symbol
34  211564_s_at     0.613 0.0004914 3.79 -0.819 1.060      PDLIM4
67    205453_at     0.613 0.0009294 3.58 -1.234 0.997       HOXB2
305 210135_s_at     0.634 0.0036540 3.09 -2.129 0.996       SHOX2
492 206201_s_at     0.634 0.0057537 2.92 -2.425 0.991       MEOX2
611   226237_at     0.650 0.0072759 2.83 -2.578 0.990      COL8A1
133   203184_at     0.613 0.0015133 3.41 -1.552 0.984        FBN2
835   228904_at     0.651 0.0102690 2.69 -2.802 0.943       HOXB3
26    237449_at     0.613 0.0004028 3.86 -0.689 0.935         SP8
11  214175_x_at     0.613 0.0001970 4.10 -0.226 0.930      PDLIM4
8     229782_at     0.613 0.0001077 4.30  0.163 0.927        RMST
                                                    Gene.title   abs
34                                        PDZ and LIM domain 4 1.060
67                                                 homeobox B2 0.997
305                                   short stature homeobox 2 0.996
492                                     mesenchyme homeobox 2 0.991
611                           collagen type VIII alpha 1 chain 0.990
133                                                fibrillin 2 0.984
835                                                homeobox B3 0.943
26                                    Sp8 transcription factor 0.935
11                                        PDZ and LIM domain 4 0.930
8   rhabdomyosarcoma 2 associated transcript (non-protein coding) 0.927
```

A look at the 10 top genes from the sorted data based on absolute log FC values shows duplicate genes for two of the probes; therefore we omit the probe with lower absolute log FC values and replace it with a new probe, or gene:

```
> top10 <- top[c(1:11),]
> top10 <- top10[-9, ]
```

In order to find these probes among the expression data set, "expressions70," we need to change the row names of both "top10" and "expressions70" to represent the probe identifiers:

```
> rownames(expressions70) <- expressions70$ID_REF
> rownames(top10) <- top10$ID
> keep <- top10$ID
> topexpressions <- expressions70[keep,]
```

Now we can change the row names into gene symbols:

```
> rownames(topexpressions) <- top10$Gene.symbol
```

In order to create our final data sets to train the classification models, we need to swap the rows and columns so each column represents a feature, that is, a significant gene, and each row represents a patient. We also need to add a new column to represent the patients' survival:

```
> data <- as.data.frame(t(topexpressions))
> data <- data[-1,]
> data <- cbind(data, survival)
> colnames(data)[11] <- "Survival"
```

We can now divide our data set into training and testing subsets to train the classification models using different algorithms:

```
> set.seed(123)
> subsets <- sample(2, nrow(data), prob=c(0.7, 0.3), replace=T)
> train <- data[subsets==1,]
> test <- data[subsets==2,]
```

Naïve Bayes' classification

We start off by training a classifier by Naïve Bayes' algorithm. From Chapter 6, we remember that this classifier performs best if the covariates are categorical and are independent from one another. In order to assess whether covariates in our data are dependent, let us examine their correlation:

```
> cor(data[,1:10])
             PDLIM4      HOXB2      SHOX2      MEOX2      COL8A1        FBN2       HOXB3
PDLIM4   1.00000000 0.54489405  0.4521434  0.4465836  0.53338247  0.07241263  0.50243033
HOXB2    0.54489405 1.00000000  0.3487733  0.4808998  0.21298808  0.02397847  0.82476049
SHOX2    0.45214338 0.34877328  1.0000000  0.6424136  0.50225684  0.17909774  0.52676031
MEOX2    0.44658364 0.48089982  0.6424136  1.0000000  0.44002907  0.22846035  0.66608533
COL8A1   0.53338247 0.21298808  0.5022568  0.4400291  1.00000000  0.25804206  0.27508283
FBN2     0.07241263 0.02397847  0.1790977  0.2284604  0.25804206  1.00000000 -0.03162782
HOXB3    0.50243033 0.82476049  0.5267603  0.6660853  0.27508283 -0.03162782  1.00000000
SP8      0.33694468 0.33175990  0.3581701  0.5049330  0.08590987 -0.04391528  0.48392246
RMST     0.25856143 0.39603914  0.3220801  0.2419625  0.18237908  0.23172055  0.38207903
ZDHHC22 -0.57128342 -0.32757465 -0.6004711 -0.4446679 -0.75007136 -0.17988482 -0.37214654
```

```
                  SP8        RMST     ZDHHC22
PDLIM4    0.33694468  0.2585614 -0.5712834
HOXB2     0.33175990  0.3960391 -0.3275746
SHOX2     0.35817014  0.3220801 -0.6004711
MEOX2     0.50493295  0.2419625 -0.4446679
COL8A1    0.08590987  0.1823791 -0.7500714
FBN2     -0.04391528  0.2317205 -0.1798848
HOXB3     0.48392246  0.3820790 -0.3721465
SP8       1.00000000  0.4741412 -0.1628854
RMST      0.47414119  1.0000000 -0.3008614
ZDHHC22 -0.16288544 -0.3008614  1.0000000
```

The output shows that covariates are not strongly correlated to one another except for a few instances, namely HOXB2 and HOXB3. Therefore the main assumption of Naïve Bayes' classifiers partly holds true. We remember from Chapter 6 that in the case of numeric variables, there are various methods to use these variables for training of Naïve Bayes' classification models. One way is for Naïve Bayes' to use mean, standard deviation, and a normal distribution formula to estimate the probabilities.

Considering these limitations in our data set, we assess the performance of a Naïve Bayes' classifier in predicting our testing observations. As all our variables are numeric, we do not need to take care of zero probabilities using Laplace smoothing. For creating the confusion matrix, we use the `confusionMatrix()` function from the "caret" package [1].

```
> library(naivebayes)
> NB <- naive_bayes(Survival~., data=train)
> predict_NB <- predict(NB, test)
Warning message:
predict.naive_bayes(): more features in the newdata are provided as there
are probability tables in the object. Calculation is performed based on
features to be found in the tables.
> ConfusionMatrix_NB <- confusionMatrix(predict_NB, test$Survival)
> ConfusionMatrix_NB
Confusion Matrix and Statistics

              Reference
Prediction     intermediate long short
  intermediate            7    2     3
  long                    1    5     1
  short                   1    0     2
```

```
Overall Statistics

               Accuracy : 0.6364
                 95% CI : (0.4066, 0.828)
    No Information Rate : 0.4091
    P-Value [Acc > NIR] : 0.02647

                  Kappa : 0.4304

 Mcnemar's Test P-Value : 0.50617

Statistics by Class:

                     Class: intermediate Class: long Class: short
Sensitivity                       0.7778      0.7143      0.33333
Specificity                       0.6154      0.8667      0.93750
Pos Pred Value                    0.5833      0.7143      0.66667
Neg Pred Value                    0.8000      0.8667      0.78947
Prevalence                        0.4091      0.3182      0.27273
Detection Rate                    0.3182      0.2273      0.09091
Detection Prevalence              0.5455      0.3182      0.13636
Balanced Accuracy                 0.6966      0.7905      0.63542
```

Our output shows that our model has an accuracy of ~60. Even though this accuracy is not high per se, the *P*-value of comparing the "NB" model with that of a map model shows that our model is considerably better than a map model. However, our predictions can be more accurate by choosing other algorithms to train our predictive model.

Logistic regression

The second classification algorithm discussed in this book, in Chapter 7, was logistic regression. Unlike Naïve Bayes', logistic regression does not have many strict assumptions. As our dependent variable is a class variable with three levels, we need to use a multinomial regression function to train our model. For this purpose, we use the `multinom()` function from the "nnet" package [2]:

```
> library(nnet)
> LRM <- multinom(Survival~., data=train)
# weights:  36 (22 variable)
initial  value 52.733390
iter  10 value 22.331097
iter  20 value 20.391454
iter  30 value 20.377672
final  value 20.377670
converged
> summary(LRM)
Call:
multinom(formula = Survival ~ ., data = train)

Coefficients:
      (Intercept)     PDLIM4     HOXB2      SHOX2      MEOX2    COL8A1       FBN2    HOXB3
long    -4.332181 -2.1148657 -6.525638 -2.7153009  3.4993903 -0.278109 -4.6812655 3.563219
short   -3.062194 -0.6314004 -1.011623  0.3641717 -0.1343919  0.117947  0.4207266 1.208332
            SP8     RMST    ZDHHC22
long  -8.9750156 4.690117  0.5302438
short -0.9550068 1.435182 -2.5178099

Std. Errors:
      (Intercept)   PDLIM4    HOXB2    SHOX2    MEOX2   COL8A1      FBN2    HOXB3       SP8
long     2.420801 1.620310 2.943210 1.602842 1.888812 1.629716 2.3799699 1.973363 4.4364235
short    1.422545 1.349249 1.419127 1.452557 1.090943 1.161120 0.8905656 1.521469 0.9653944
          RMST  ZDHHC22
long  2.295124 2.338145
short 1.406470 1.514357


Residual Deviance: 40.75534
AIC: 84.75534
> predict_LRM <- predict(LRM, test, type="class")
> ConfusionMatrix_LRM <- confusionMatrix(predict_LRM, test$Survival)
> ConfusionMatrix_LRM
Confusion Matrix and Statistics


              Reference
Prediction     intermediate long short
  intermediate            7    0     5
  long                    2    7     1
  short                   0    0     0
```

```
Overall Statistics

               Accuracy : 0.6364
                 95% CI : (0.4066, 0.828)
    No Information Rate : 0.4091
    P-Value [Acc > NIR] : 0.02647

                  Kappa : 0.4248

 Mcnemar's Test P-Value : 0.04601

Statistics by Class:

                     Class: intermediate Class: long Class: short
Sensitivity                       0.7778      1.0000       0.0000
Specificity                       0.6154      0.8000       1.0000
Pos Pred Value                    0.5833      0.7000          NaN
Neg Pred Value                    0.8000      1.0000       0.7273
Prevalence                        0.4091      0.3182       0.2727
Detection Rate                    0.3182      0.3182       0.0000
Detection Prevalence              0.5455      0.4545       0.0000
Balanced Accuracy                 0.6966      0.9000       0.5000
```

Even though the confusion matrices of the LRM and NB classifiers are showing different patterns of misclassification of data, the percentage of accuracy, hence the P-values, of the two models is the same in this instance. Our data are more concordant with the assumptions of multinomial regression than those of Naïve Bayes' classifier; however, logistic regression may not be a better algorithm to train a classifier using these data. In addition to a slightly higher Kappa coefficient of the NB model, a look at the "Statistics by class" section of the confusion matrix output of the two models shows that logistic regression has zero sensitivity for the class "short" of the observations. Therefore, in addition to the algorithm used to train a model, there are several other factors that need to be considered when choosing one model over the other.

Linear and quadratic discriminant analysis

Now let us see if quadratic or linear discriminant analysis (QDA and LDA, respectively) can outperform the classifiers created thus far in this chapter. From Chapter 8, we remember that QDA and LDA have their own assumptions; however, an important aspect that determines which of these two algorithms must be used is homogeneity of variance in independent variables for each class of the dependent variable. For this purpose, we used Levene's test from the "car" package [3].

```
> library(car)
> leveneTest(data$PDLIM4, data$Survival, center=mean)
Levene's Test for Homogeneity of Variance (center = mean)
      Df F value Pr(>F)
group  2  0.2819 0.7552
      67
> leveneTest(data$HOXB2, data$Survival, center=mean)
Levene's Test for Homogeneity of Variance (center = mean)
      Df F value Pr(>F)
group  2  0.5618 0.5728
      67
> leveneTest(data$SHOX2, data$Survival, center=mean)
Levene's Test for Homogeneity of Variance (center = mean)
      Df F value  Pr(>F)
group  2  6.6194 0.00238 **
      67
---
Signif. codes:  0 '***' 0.001 '**' 0.01 '*' 0.05 '.' 0.1 ' ' 1
> leveneTest(data$MEOX2, data$Survival, center=mean)
Levene's Test for Homogeneity of Variance (center = mean)
      Df F value  Pr(>F)
group  2  3.7231 0.02929 *
      67
---
Signif. codes:  0 '***' 0.001 '**' 0.01 '*' 0.05 '.' 0.1 ' ' 1
> leveneTest(data$COL8A1, data$Survival, center=mean)
Levene's Test for Homogeneity of Variance (center = mean)
      Df F value  Pr(>F)
group  2  2.5093 0.08894 .
      67
---
```

```
Signif. codes:  0 '***' 0.001 '**' 0.01 '*' 0.05 '.' 0.1 ' ' 1
> leveneTest(data$FBN2, data$Survival, center=mean)
Levene's Test for Homogeneity of Variance (center = mean)
      Df F value Pr(>F)
group  2  0.2944 0.7459
      67
> leveneTest(data$HOXB3, data$Survival, center=mean)
Levene's Test for Homogeneity of Variance (center = mean)
      Df F value Pr(>F)
group  2  1.5185 0.2265
      67
> leveneTest(data$SP8, data$Survival, center=mean)
Levene's Test for Homogeneity of Variance (center = mean)
      Df F value    Pr(>F)
group  2  18.883 3.134e-07 ***
      67
---
Signif. codes:  0 '***' 0.001 '**' 0.01 '*' 0.05 '.' 0.1 ' ' 1
> leveneTest(data$RMST, data$Survival, center=mean)
Levene's Test for Homogeneity of Variance (center = mean)
      Df F value Pr(>F)
group  2  0.7458 0.4782
      67
> leveneTest(data$ZDHHC22, data$Survival, center=mean)
Levene's Test for Homogeneity of Variance (center = mean)
      Df F value Pr(>F)
group  2  0.4013  0.671
      67
```

The assumption of homogeneity of variance of independent variables is met for most of the variables. In order to have an idea of distribution of each independent variable, we plot the distributions. For better visualization, let us plot the variables. Even though there are several methods to plot a data distribution in R, in order to use fewer lines of programming, we use the `pairs.panels( )` function from the "psych" package [4]. These plots have the advantage of showing an association of different variables with one another, in addition to showing the extent to which a class of observations can be determined based on each independent variable. For better visualization, the first five independent variables are demonstrated in one plot, and the second five variables of the data are demonstrated in a separate plot.

```
> plot1 <- pairs.panels(data[1:5],bg=c("red","yellow","blue")[data$Survival],
+            pch=21,)
> plot2 <-
pairs.panels(data[6:10],bg=c("red","yellow","blue")[data$Survival],
+                      pch=21,)
```

Fig. 14.1 shows that data are not normally distributed for each variable. Even though this will compromise the performance of discriminant-based algorithms to some extent, we can still use these

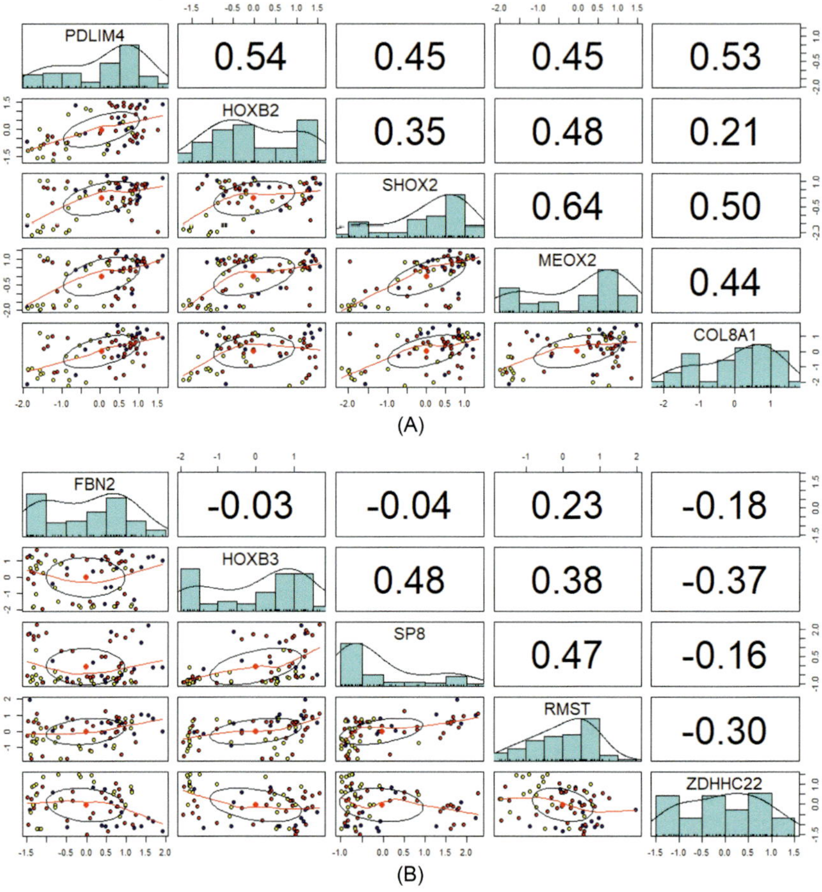

FIGURE 14.1 (A) Distribution of data for each independent variable. (B) Distribution of data for each independent variable.

algorithms for training our classifiers. As some of the independent variables do not have homogeneous variances for each class of dependent variables, we use QDA over LDA for our model.

We remember from Chapter 8 that we need to preprocess our data in order to standardize them before training our model. For this purpose, we use `preprocess()` from the "caret" package.

```
> preprocessParams <- preProcess(data[,1:11], method=c("range"))
> print(preprocessParams)
Created from 70 samples and 11 variables


Pre-processing:
  - ignored (1)
  - re-scaling to [0, 1] (10)
> transformed <- predict(preprocessParams, data[,1:11])
```

The `preprocess()` function automatically ignores the categorical variables. Now that our data have been standardized, we divide these rescaled data into training and testing subsets.

```
> set.seed(123)
> subsets <- sample(2, nrow(transformed), prob=c(0.7, 0.3), replace=T)
> transformedtrain <- transformed[subsets==1,]
> transformedtest <- transformed[subsets==2,]
```

Now our data are ready to train the QDA classifier. For this purpose, we use the `qda()` function from the "MASS" package [2]:

```
> QDA <- qda(Survival~., data=transformedtrain)
Error in qda.default(x, grouping, ...) :
  some group is too small for 'qda'
```

In the "MASS" package, whenever the number of observations in each class of dependent variables is equal to or smaller than the number of independent variables used to train the model, the function returns an error. In our transformed training data, the number of observations from the class "short" is 10, which is equal to the number of independent variables:

```
> sum(transformedtrain$Survival=="long")
[1] 16
> sum(transformedtrain$Survival=="short")
[1] 10
> sum(transformedtrain$Survival=="intermediate")
[1] 22
```

Therefore we need to decrease the number of predictors in training our model. Even though reducing this number to any number smaller than 10 will resolve the error, we opt to decrease the number of predictors to as low as three. As discussed in Chapter 5, there are several ways to choose certain features. One of these methods is to find variables that affect the survival the most. For this purpose, we choose the three variables that have the highest absolute coefficient values in the summary of our LRM model.

```
> QDA <- qda(Survival~ HOXB2 + SP8 + FBN2, data=transformedtrain)
> predict_QDA <- predict(QDA, transformedtest, type="prob")
> ConfusionMatrix_QDA <- confusionMatrix(predict_QDA$class,
transformedtest$Survival)
> ConfusionMatrix_QDA
Confusion Matrix and Statistics

              Reference
Prediction     intermediate long short
  intermediate            7    1     4
  long                    2    6     1
  short                   0    0     1

Overall Statistics

               Accuracy : 0.6364
                 95% CI : (0.4066, 0.828)
    No Information Rate : 0.4091
    P-Value [Acc > NIR] : 0.02647

                  Kappa : 0.4267

 Mcnemar's Test P-Value : 0.14895
```

```
Statistics by Class:

                     Class: intermediate Class: long Class: short
Sensitivity                       0.7778      0.8571      0.16667
Specificity                       0.6154      0.8000      1.00000
Pos Pred Value                    0.5833      0.6667      1.00000
Neg Pred Value                    0.8000      0.9231      0.76190
Prevalence                        0.4091      0.3182      0.27273
Detection Rate                    0.3182      0.2727      0.04545
Detection Prevalence              0.5455      0.4091      0.04545
Balanced Accuracy                 0.6966      0.8286      0.58333
```

The accuracy of the QDA model is similar to the previous models; however, it must be noted that the number of predictors in the QDA model is far fewer than those of the NB and LRM models. The effects of fewer predictors can act as a double-edged sword: Even though the ratio of observations to predictors increases, which allows better learning and fitting of the model to the observations, we are missing predictors that can potentially increase the performance of the model by providing useful information.

Support vector machine

Support vector machine (SVM) classifiers try to find boundaries that can best distinguish data points based on their categories. Unlike linear algorithms such as logistic regression, the decision boundary is not confined to being linear for SVM, which can improve the performance of the model, specifically in cases where our data points do not follow a linear trend. In order to train our SVM classifier, similar to Chapter 9, we use the "e1071" package [5]:

```
> library(e1071)
> SVM <- svm(Survival~., data=train)
> predict_SVM <- predict(SVM, test)
> ConfusionMatrix_SVM <- confusionMatrix(predict_SVM, test$Survival)
> ConfusionMatrix_SVM
Confusion Matrix and Statistics
```

```
              Reference
Prediction     intermediate long short
  intermediate            9    2     4
  long                    0    5     1
  short                   0    0     1

Overall Statistics

               Accuracy : 0.6818
                 95% CI : (0.4513, 0.8614)
    No Information Rate : 0.4091
    P-Value [Acc > NIR] : 0.008992

                  Kappa : 0.4884

 Mcnemar's Test P-Value : 0.071898

Statistics by Class:

                     Class: intermediate Class: long Class: short
Sensitivity                       1.0000      0.7143      0.16667
Specificity                       0.5385      0.9333      1.00000
Pos Pred Value                    0.6000      0.8333      1.00000
Neg Pred Value                    1.0000      0.8750      0.76190
Prevalence                        0.4091      0.3182      0.27273
Detection Rate                    0.4091      0.2273      0.04545
Detection Prevalence              0.6818      0.2727      0.04545
Balanced Accuracy                 0.7692      0.8238      0.58333
```

As could be predicted, SVM outperformed linear-based models, as well as other models created thus far in this chapter. In addition to accuracy, there are other reasons such as increased Kappa coefficient, as well as no misclassification of observations belonging to the "intermediate" category, that make SVM a more dependable model compared to NB, LRM, and QDA.

Decision trees

Decision trees are among the several algorithms that can be used for both classification and regression problems. In Chapter 10, we learnt how to create a decision tree classifier using the "party" package [6]. In this chapter, we learn how to train decision trees using the "rpart" and "rpart.plot" packages [7,8], and how to tune the parameters of our model to prevent overfitting the model on the training data, which can diminish its performance on unseen data.

We start by installing and calling the required packages:

```
> install.packages("rpart")
> install.packages("rpart")
> library(rpart)
> install.packages("rpart.plot")
> install.packages("rpart.plot")
> library(rpart.plot)
```

Now we can train our decision tree based on our training data. Even though all arguments are described in detail in the documentation of the `rpart()` function, we will overview some of these arguments and parameters. In order to split our tree based on retrieved information, we need to set the "parms" argument to "information"; otherwise, the Gini index will be used as default for splitting branches. The other important factor is complexity parameter or "cp." This parameter determines the minimum improvement in the model's fit that we wish to observe at each split, and if the inclusion of a variable or splitting of a node does not increase the model's fit by at least a factor of "cp," then the split or inclusion of the variable does not occur. Two other factors that we will determine in training our model are "minsplit" and "minbucket," in order to determine the minimum number of observations in a node for split to occur, and the minimum number of observations in a terminal node in order for a split to occur. We can also determine to what extent we want to split our tree in terms of levels of splitting by determining the "maxdepth."

In order to be able to prune our tree, we want to generate very large numbers of splitting in our tree, and let our tree grow to its potential. In order to do so, we need to set "cp" to a very small number. Then, we can find the optimal "cp" to prune the tree to prevent overfitting of the tree on the training data.

```
> DT <- rpart(Survival~., data=data,
+             method="class", parms = list(split="information"),
+             control = rpart.control(cp=0.0000001, minsplit = 5, minbucket =
2, maxdepth = 10 ))
```

We can now plot (Fig. 14.2) this decision tree using the `rpart.plot()` function:

```
> rpart.plot(DT)
```

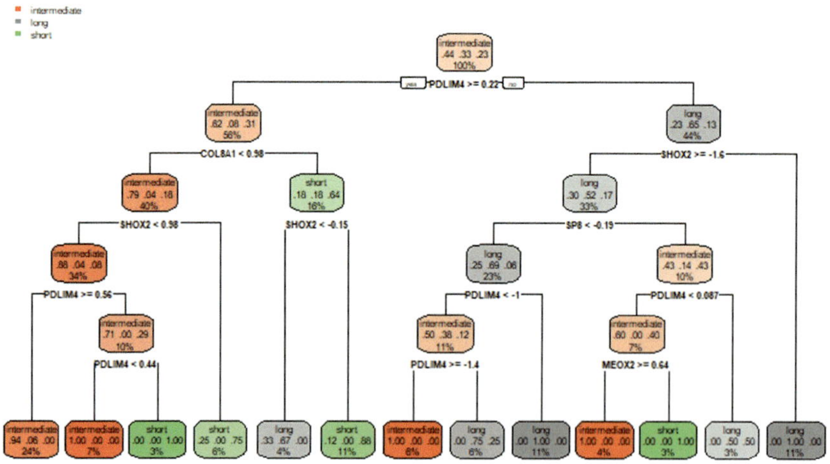

FIGURE 14.2 Plot of the decision tree with a very low complexity parameter.

In order to find the optimal "cp," we can either plot "cp" against the errors in cross-validation (Fig. 14.3) or we can use the `printcp()` function of the "rpart" package.

```
> plotcp(DT)
> printcp(DT)

Classification tree:
rpart(formula = Survival ~ ., data = data, method = "class",
    parms = list(split = "information"), control = rpart.control(cp = 1e-07,
        minsplit = 5, minbucket = 2, maxdepth = 10))

Variables actually used in tree construction:
[1] COL8A1 MEOX2  PDLIM4 SHOX2  SP8

Root node error: 39/70 = 0.55714

n= 70

         CP nsplit rel error  xerror    xstd
1 0.3333333      0   1.00000 1.00000 0.10656
2 0.1282051      1   0.66667 0.69231 0.10442
3 0.0512821      2   0.53846 0.76923 0.10616
4 0.0384615      4   0.43590 0.89744 0.10726
5 0.0256410     10   0.20513 0.92308 0.10722
6 0.0000001     12   0.15385 0.87179 0.10722
```

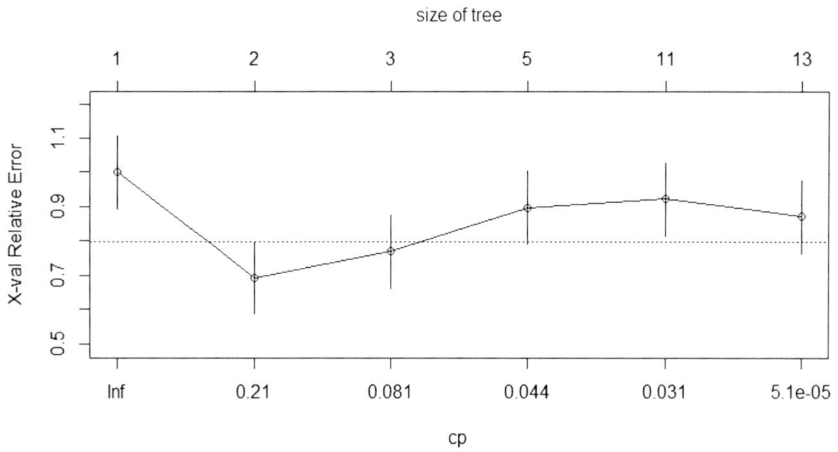

FIGURE 14.3 Plot of the complexity parameter against cross-validation relative error.

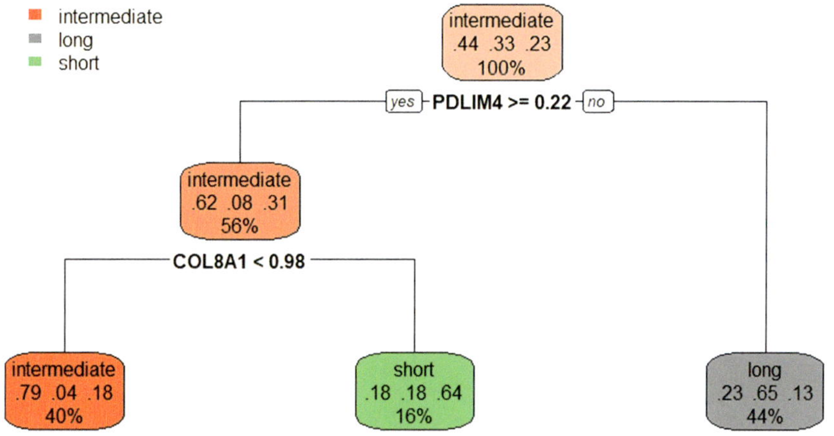

FIGURE 14.4 Plot of the pruned decision tree.

In order to find the optimal value for "cp" to prune our decision tree, we must find the "cp" value that resulted in the minimum cross-validation error, denoted by "xerror." For our decision tree, the corresponding "cp" value is 0.1282051. In order to find the optimal decision tree and test its accuracy using the testing subset, we create a new decision tree using the `prune()` function of the "rpart" package:

```
> pruned_DT <- prune(DT, cp=0.1282051)
```

Now we can plot the pruned decision tree to evaluate the final decision tree (Fig. 14.4).

```
> rpart.plot(pruned_DT)
```

We can now predict our test data using the pruned decision tree model:

```
> predict_DT <- predict(pruned_DT, test)
> ConfusionMatrix_DT <- confusionMatrix(predict_NB, test$Survival)
> ConfusionMatrix_DT
Confusion Matrix and Statistics

              Reference
Prediction     intermediate long short
  intermediate            7    2     3
  long                    1    5     1
  short                   1    0     2

Overall Statistics

               Accuracy : 0.6364
                 95% CI : (0.4066, 0.828)
    No Information Rate : 0.4091
    P-Value [Acc > NIR] : 0.02647

                  Kappa : 0.4304

 Mcnemar's Test P-Value : 0.50617

Statistics by Class:

                     Class: intermediate Class: long Class: short
Sensitivity                       0.7778      0.7143      0.33333
Specificity                       0.6154      0.8667      0.93750
Pos Pred Value                    0.5833      0.7143      0.66667
Neg Pred Value                    0.8000      0.8667      0.78947
Prevalence                        0.4091      0.3182      0.27273
Detection Rate                    0.3182      0.2273      0.09091
Detection Prevalence              0.5455      0.3182      0.13636
Balanced Accuracy                 0.6966      0.7905      0.63542
```

Decision tree model's performance is similar to that of NB, LRM, and QDA. However, this must be regarded in light of the fact that the decision tree only used four variables for making predictions.

Random forest

Similar to decision trees, random forests are powerful algorithms that can be used for both classification and regression problems. However, they have certain advantages over decision trees. Unlike decision trees, the risk of overfitting on the training data is lower in random forests. Furthermore, random forests are better at handling a large number of features, and can even be used for feature selection.

In Chapter 11, we learnt about principles of training random forest classifiers and regression models. Now we implement similar methods for creating random forest classifiers. In addition, we learn how to tune our model parameters to improve the model's performance and decrease computational costs for developing random forest models. We use the "randomForest" package [9] for making our random forest classifiers.

```
> library(randomForest)
```

As a random forest, evident from its name, randomly selects obser-vartions during bootstrapping, we need to fix this effect of randomization to generate reproducible results.

```
> set.seed(123)
```

Now we can train our model. In Chapter 11, we discussed that for random forest classifiers, "mtry," which denotes the number of variables randomly sampled as candidates at each split, is set to a square root of the number of features as default. For the number of trees generated through bootstrapping, we need to choose a large number; here, we choose this number to be 500. This number can be adjusted during the tuning process to decrease temporal and computational costs of random forest models.

```
> RF <- randomForest(Survival~., data=train, ntree=500)
> print(RF)

Call:
 randomForest(formula = Survival ~ ., data = train, ntree = 500)
               Type of random forest: classification
                     Number of trees: 500
No. of variables tried at each split: 3
```

```
        OOB estimate of  error rate: 50%
Confusion matrix:
             intermediate long short class.error
intermediate           12    8     2   0.4545455
long                    8    7     1   0.5625000
short                   4    1     5   0.5000000
```

The summary of the model shows a high out-of-bag error, which shows how the model predicts the part of training data that was not included in the bootstrapping. Furthermore, the classification error shown in the confusion matrix is high. Let us evaluate how our model performs in predicting a class of observations in the testing subset.

```
> predict_RF <- predict(RF, test)
> ConfusionMatrix_RF <- confusionMatrix(predict_RF, test$Survival)
> ConfusionMatrix_RF
Confusion Matrix and Statistics

              Reference
Prediction     intermediate long short
  intermediate            9    2     5
  long                    0    5     1
  short                   0    0     0

Overall Statistics

               Accuracy : 0.6364
                 95% CI : (0.4066, 0.828)
    No Information Rate : 0.4091
    P-Value [Acc > NIR] : 0.02647

                  Kappa : 0.4094

 Mcnemar's Test P-Value : 0.04601
```

```
Statistics by Class:

                     Class: intermediate Class: long Class: short
Sensitivity                       1.0000      0.7143       0.0000
Specificity                       0.4615      0.9333       1.0000
Pos Pred Value                    0.5625      0.8333          NaN
Neg Pred Value                    1.0000      0.8750       0.7273
Prevalence                        0.4091      0.3182       0.2727
Detection Rate                    0.4091      0.2273       0.0000
Detection Prevalence              0.7273      0.2727       0.0000
Balanced Accuracy                 0.7308      0.8238       0.5000
```

Performance of our random forest model is similar to some of the previous classifiers in terms of accuracy percentage; however, a random forest classifier demonstrates a poor performance regarding the types of misclassifications and is inclined toward predicting certain classes.

Let us see how we can change the parameters of our model in order to improve these statistics. One of the parameters of the model that may not directly affect its predictions but can lower computational costs of the model is the number of trees generated by the model. In order to decrease this number in a way that does not affect the model's performance, we need to plot the number of trees against the error rate of the model (Fig. 14.5).

```
> plot(RF)
```

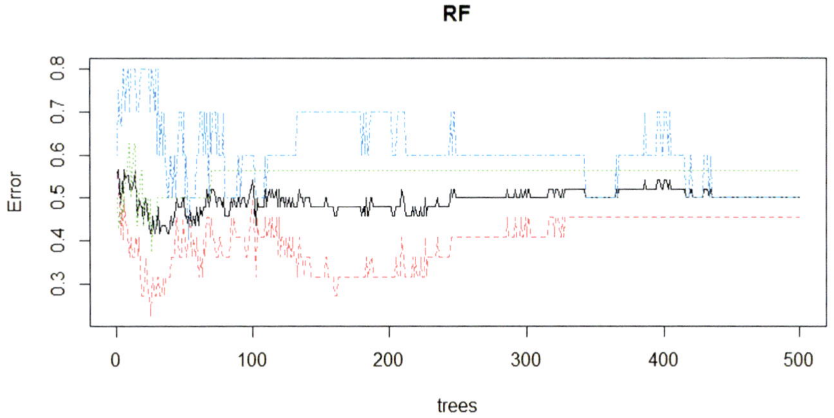

FIGURE 14.5 Plot of the number of trees in the random forest against the model's error.

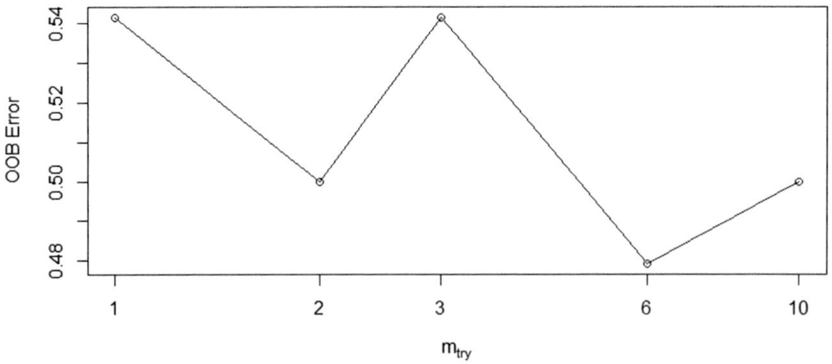

FIGURE 14.6 Effect of different "mtry" values on the model's out-of-bag error.

Even though the error rate fluctuates, we can successfully decrease the number of trees by 400 without compromising the model's performance. There are other parameters that can be changed. In order to set these parameters, we use the `tuneRF()` function of the "randomForest" package [9]. We overview some of the important arguments of this function for our learning purposes.

To tune our model, we choose a small improvement in the out-of-bag error for the model to keep trying various parameters. If this improvement is not made, the model will stop iterations. We can also decrease the number of trees to 400, as it does not affect the model's performance. We also plot the effect of different "mtry" values on the error rate of our model (Fig. 14.6), and keep track of these effects by setting the "trace" argument to true.

```
> set.seed(123)
> tunedRF <- tuneRF(train[,-11], train[,11],
+                  ntreeTry = 400, improve = 0.04,
+                  plot= T, trace = T)
mtry = 3  OOB error = 54.17%
Searching left ...
mtry = 2    OOB error = 50%
0.07692308 0.04
mtry = 1    OOB error = 54.17%
-0.08333333 0.04
Searching right ...
mtry = 6    OOB error = 47.92%
0.04166667 0.04
mtry = 10   OOB error = 50%
-0.04347826 0.04
```

We can see that the lowest out-of-bag error is achieved with mtry = 6. We can now implement these findings in modifying our model parameters.

```
> set.seed(123)
> modified_RF <- randomForest(Survival~., data=train, ntree=400, mtry=6)
> print(modified_RF)

Call:
 randomForest(formula = Survival ~ ., data = train, ntree = 400,     mtry = 6)
               Type of random forest: classification
                     Number of trees: 400
No. of variables tried at each split: 6

        OOB estimate of  error rate: 47.92%
Confusion matrix:
             intermediate long short class.error
intermediate           13    5     4   0.4090909
long                    7    8     1   0.5000000
short                   5    1     4   0.6000000
```

Even though the improvement in the out-of-bag error is not remarkable, the improvement in the model's classifications can be perceivable.

```
> predict_mRF <- predict(modified_RF, test)
> ConfusionMatrix_mRF <- confusionMatrix(predict_mRF, test$Survival)
> ConfusionMatrix_mRF
Confusion Matrix and Statistics

              Reference
Prediction     intermediate long short
  intermediate            9    1     5
  long                    0    6     1
  short                   0    0     0
```

```
Overall Statistics

               Accuracy : 0.6818
                 95% CI : (0.4513, 0.8614)
    No Information Rate : 0.4091
    P-Value [Acc > NIR] : 0.008992

                  Kappa : 0.4867

 Mcnemar's Test P-Value : 0.071898

Statistics by Class:

                     Class: intermediate Class: long Class: short
Sensitivity                       1.0000      0.8571       0.0000
Specificity                       0.5385      0.9333       1.0000
Pos Pred Value                    0.6000      0.8571          NaN
Neg Pred Value                    1.0000      0.9333       0.7273
Prevalence                        0.4091      0.3182       0.2727
Detection Rate                    0.4091      0.2727       0.0000
Detection Prevalence              0.6818      0.3182       0.0000
Balanced Accuracy                 0.7692      0.8952       0.5000
```

Even though our model's accuracy has increased in percentage, the patterns of misclassifications are not improved. Feature selection, as discussed in Chapter 11, may improve the model's performance as the proportion of observations to features increases. Using feature selection for improving the model's performance is left to interested readers.

K-nearest neighbors

Similar to many other algorithms discussed in this book, K-nearest neighbors (KNNs) algorithms can be used to create both classification and regression models. In this section, we create a KNN classifier using the `train()` function of the "caret" package.

In KNN, similar to random forest, and some other algorithms discussed in this book, we need to eliminate the effect of randomization in order to attain reproducible results. Arguments of the `train()` function that are important for creating a KNN model have been discussed in Chapter 12. We can choose for our algorithm to try more *K* values to find the optimum *K* value; however, this will result in increased computational costs and time for training the model. The same holds true for a higher number of cross-validation groups.

```
> set.seed(1234)
> KNN <- train(Survival~., data=train,
+                  method="knn",
+                  trControl=trainControl("cv", number=5),
+                  preProcess=c("scale", "center"),
+                  tuneLength=30)
There were 50 or more warnings (use warnings() to see the first 50)
```

As discussed in Chapter 12, the warnings returned are due to the fact that values that are being tested for *K* are greater than the number of observations in the training data. We now move on to compare the accuracy of the KNN predictions for the test data with other models created in this chapter.

```
> predict_KNN <- predict(KNN, test)
> ConfusionMatrix_KNN <- confusionMatrix(predict_KNN, test$Survival)
> ConfusionMatrix_KNN
Confusion Matrix and Statistics

              Reference
Prediction     intermediate long short
  intermediate            8    2     4
  long                    1    5     1
  short                   0    0     1

Overall Statistics

               Accuracy : 0.6364
                 95% CI : (0.4066, 0.828)
    No Information Rate : 0.4091
    P-Value [Acc > NIR] : 0.02647

                  Kappa : 0.4191

 Mcnemar's Test P-Value : 0.14895
```

```
Statistics by Class:

                     Class: intermediate Class: long Class: short
Sensitivity                       0.8889      0.7143      0.16667
Specificity                       0.5385      0.8667      1.00000
Pos Pred Value                    0.5714      0.7143      1.00000
Neg Pred Value                    0.8750      0.8667      0.76190
Prevalence                        0.4091      0.3182      0.27273
Detection Rate                    0.3636      0.2273      0.04545
Detection Prevalence              0.6364      0.3182      0.04545
Balanced Accuracy                 0.7137      0.7905      0.58333
```

The accuracy of the model is comparable to the majority of the models created in this chapter; however, a look at the statistics by class section of the confusion matrix summary shows that this model performs better than some other models, such as the random forest classifier, in terms of trends in misclassification. These factors must be considered when choosing one machine learning algorithm over another.

Neural networks

As discussed in Chapter 13, neural networks are powerful algorithms that can be used for both classification and regression problems; however, their use must be reserved for appropriate data sets. In this chapter, for our learning purposes, we create neural network classifiers with our data; however, it must be noted that several factors make neural networks not ideal for making predictions on our data set. One of these factors is the size of our data set; neural networks are best reserved for large data sets where they can identify features and hidden patterns. The other factor is that neural networks act as black boxes; therefore, even if they find certain patterns in our data, their results are not easily interpretable. An advantage that neural networks have is that they can easily work with a high number of features, which can be useful for biological data. Even though we can take benefit from this feature of neural networks for our model and increase the number of features used to train the data, we leave this to interested audience and move on with training our neural network classifiers using the 10 features used for most of the other models in this chapter.

We use the `neuralnet()` function of the "neuralnet" package [10] for training our model. But, before training the model, we need to standardize our testing and training data so the weights assigned to each feature are not biased.

```
> scaledtrain <- as.data.frame(scale(train[,-11], center = T, scale = T))
> scaledtrain <- cbind(scaledtrain, train$Survival)
> colnames(scaledtrain)[11] <- "Survival"
> scaledtest <- as.data.frame(scale(test[,-11], center = T, scale = T))
> scaledtest <- cbind(scaledtest, test$Survival)
> colnames(scaledtest)[11] <- "Survival"
```

We can now move on to training the model. We remember from Chapter 13 that, ideally, the number of neurons in the hidden layer is a number between the number of the features and the number of nodes in the output layer. Therefore we choose to have five neurons in the hidden layer; however, this number can be altered. For the activation function, we use a logistic function.

```
> library(neuralnet)
> set.seed(123)
> NN1 <- neuralnet(Survival~., data=scaledtrain,
+                   hidden=5, act.fct = "logistic",
+                   linear.output = F, err.fct="ce", threshold = 0.01)
```

Features of the model that can be used for making assumptions regarding its performance have been discussed in Chapter 13. For comparison purposes, we move on to predicting observations in the testing subset using an NN1 classifier. As the returned values are probabilities, we need to make some alterations in our prediction output before using them in the `confusionMatrix()` function.

```
> predict_NN=predict(NN1, test)
> Pred_NN <- ifelse(predict_NN > 0.5, 1, 0)
> Pred_NN <- as.data.frame(Pred_NN)
> Pred_NN$Survival[Pred_NN$V1==1]="short"
> Pred_NN$Survival[Pred_NN$V2==1]="intermediate"
> Pred_NN$Survival[Pred_NN$V3==1]="long"
> Pred_NN$Survival <- as.factor(Pred_NN$Survival)
> Pred_NN <- as.data.frame(Pred_NN)
> ConfusionMatrix_NN <- confusionMatrix(Pred_NN$Survival,
scaledtest$Survival)
> ConfusionMatrix_NN
Confusion Matrix and Statistics


              Reference
Prediction     intermediate long short
  intermediate            1    5     1
  long                    0    0     2
  short                   7    2     3
```

```
Overall Statistics

               Accuracy : 0.1905
                 95% CI : (0.0545, 0.4191)
    No Information Rate : 0.381
    P-Value [Acc > NIR] : 0.98294

                  Kappa : -0.194

 Mcnemar's Test P-Value : 0.02333

Statistics by Class:

                     Class: intermediate Class: long Class: short
Sensitivity                      0.12500     0.00000       0.5000
Specificity                      0.53846     0.85714       0.4000
Pos Pred Value                   0.14286     0.00000       0.2500
Neg Pred Value                   0.50000     0.63158       0.6667
Prevalence                       0.38095     0.33333       0.2857
Detection Rate                   0.04762     0.00000       0.1429
Detection Prevalence             0.33333     0.09524       0.5714
Balanced Accuracy                0.33173     0.42857       0.4500
```

All statistics regarding the performance of our neural network classifiers reflect a very poor performance. Even though changing certain parameters of the model such as activation function or number of features used to train the model, may improve its performance, these trends indicate that neural networks are not ideal algorithms for our data set for several reasons, some of which were discussed earlier. Interested audience is encouraged to try different model parameters and study their effect on the model's accuracy.

Regression models

We now move on to creating regression models using the data obtained from GSE83300. In order to find features for training our model, which are the genes that have highest log fold change of expression, we compare the gene expression of patients with long (>36 months) and short (<12 months) survival. As our data set has only 50 observations, we choose only five features for training our regression models.

We will be making regression models using linear regression, SVM, decision tree, random forest, KNN, and neural networks. Even though there are several aspects to be considered for choosing one model over another to make predictions, we choose root mean squared error (RMSE) to compare the performances of models in making predictions.

Let us prepare our data set following similar steps to preparing the data set for classification models. Patients characteristics are obtained from GSE83300 on GEO. GEO2R is used to find the comparison statistics between the long and short survival groups and the results are stored as "GEO2R_reg." Patients' expression profiles are called "expressions" in the following lines of code.

```
> GEO2R_reg$abs <- abs(GEO2R_reg$logFC)
> GEO2R_reg$abs <- abs(GEO2R_reg$logFC)
> top_reg <- GEO2R_reg[order(GEO2R_reg$abs, decreasing=T),]
> top5 <- top_reg[c(1:5),]
> rownames(top5) <- top5$ID
> keep <- top5$ID
> top5expressions <- expressions[keep,]
> rownames(top5expressions) <- top5$Gene.symbol
> data <- as.data.frame(t(top5expressions))
> characteristics <- read.delim("patient characteristics.txt")
> Survival <- as.data.frame(characteristics$OS)
> data <- cbind(data, Survival)
> colnames(data)[6] <- "Survival"
```

Now our data set is ready to be divided into training and testing subsets.

```
> set.seed(123)
> subsets <- sample(2, nrow(reg_data), prob=c(0.7, 0.3), replace=T)
> reg_train <- reg_data[subsets==1,]
> reg_test <- reg_data[subsets==2,]
```

Linear regression

From Chapter 7, we remember that a linear regression algorithm has several assumptions. In order to understand whether our observations follow a linear trend, we plot the variables using the `pairs.panels( )` function (Fig. 14.7). The fitted line on each for each of the variables in Fig. 14.7 shows that some of the variables do not follow a linear trend. For the rest of the assumptions, we need to create our linear regression model first.

```
> pairs.panels(reg_data)
> LR <- lm(Survival~., data=reg_train)
> summary(LR)

Call:
lm(formula = Survival ~ ., data = reg_train)

Residuals:
    Min      1Q  Median      3Q     Max
-14.022  -6.015  -1.039   5.320  17.665

Coefficients:
            Estimate Std. Error t value Pr(>|t|)
(Intercept)  37.4475    11.3860   3.289  0.00264 **
SAA1         -0.3923     0.6766  -0.580  0.56651
CHI3L2       -1.7662     1.0586  -1.668  0.10602
LTF           1.5833     0.9208   1.719  0.09619 .
CHI3L1       -1.0697     1.1684  -0.916  0.36745
PRAME         1.0681     0.5716   1.869  0.07180 .
---
Signif. codes:  0 '***' 0.001 '**' 0.01 '*' 0.05 '.' 0.1 ' ' 1

Residual standard error: 8.981 on 29 degrees of freedom
Multiple R-squared:  0.3474,  Adjusted R-squared:  0.2348
F-statistic: 3.087 on 5 and 29 DF,  p-value: 0.02356
```

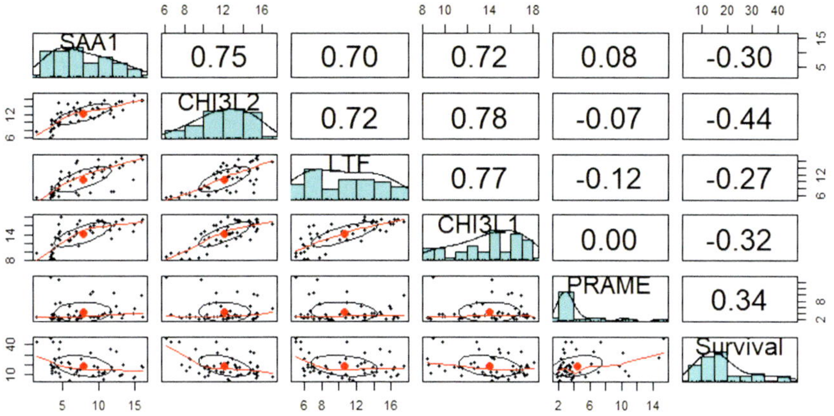

FIGURE 14.7 Plot of variables from regression data sets.

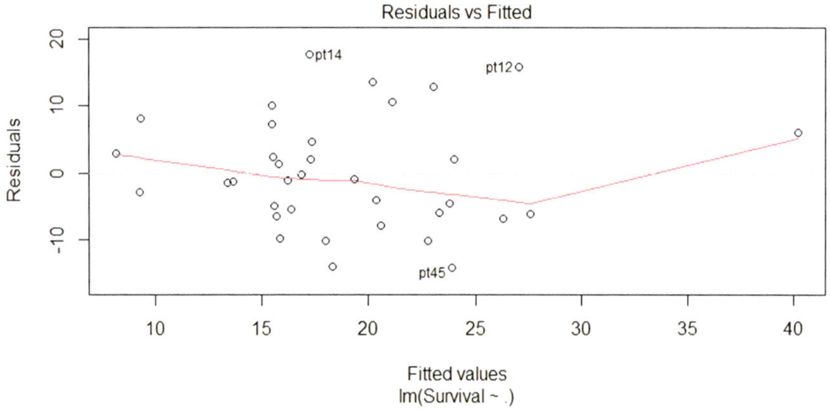

FIGURE 14.8 Diagnostic plot of residuals versus fitted values. As the fit line (red line) is not a straight, horizontal line, the data do not perfectly follow the linearity assumption.

Statistics from the model's summary are not promising due to small adjusted R-squared. Let us see if our data follow the assumptions of the linear regression model. For this model, we use the `plot()` function to plot the model. This function produces several plots. Figs. 14.8 and 14.9 show two of these plots, which demonstrate whether our data follow the assumptions. From these

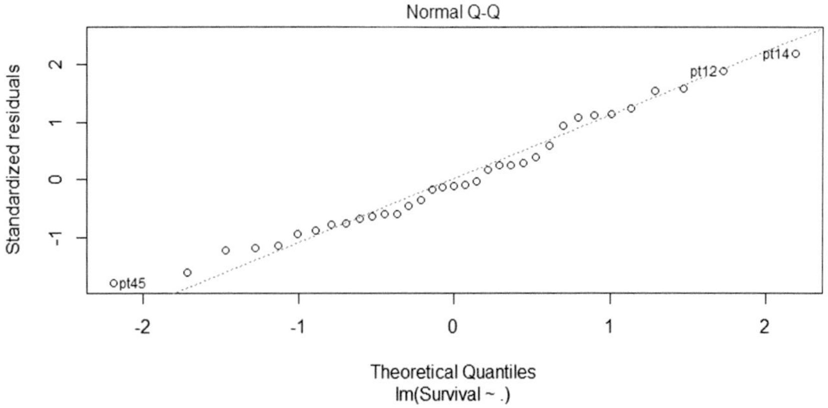

FIGURE 14.9 Diagnostic Q–Q plot, which shows that residuals do not perfectly follow the normal distribution, as there are some levels of deviation of residuals from the diagonal line.

figures, we can understand that our data do not perfectly match the assumptions of a linear regression model, which is reflected in the adjusted *R*-squared of the model. In order to have a better idea of the model's predictions, let us predict the observations in the test value and calculate the RMSE of the model for this prediction. For this purpose, we use the `rmse()` function of the "Metrics" package [11].

```
> library(Metrics)
> predict_LR <- predict(LR, reg_test)
> RMSE_LR <- rmse(predict_LR, reg_test$Survival)
> RMSE_LR
[1] 10.51095
```

Support vector regression

We now move on to predicting patients' survival in months using the SVM algorithm. The principles of creating support vector regression models are similar to those of SVM classifiers, and we use the `svm()` function from the "e1071" package.

```
> library(e1071)
> SVR <- svm(Survival~., data=reg_train)
> summary(SVR)

Call:
svm(formula = Survival ~ ., data = reg_train)


Parameters:
   SVM-Type:  eps-regression
 SVM-Kernel:  radial
       cost:  1
      gamma:  0.2
    epsilon:  0.1


Number of Support Vectors:  31
```

Out of the 35 observations in the training data set, 31 were used as support vectors to train the model and make decision boundaries. In order to compare the performance of SVR with linear regression, we calculate the RMSE for the model.

```
> predict_SVR <- predict(SVR, reg_test)
> RMSE_SVR <- rmse(predict_SVR, reg_test$Survival)
> RMSE_SVR
[1] 10.96647
```

Even though the RMSE values for the LR and SVR models are comparable, LR shows a slightly better performance, which can be justified by the approximately linear trend of the data and higher number of observations used by LR to make predictions.

Decision trees for regression

We now implement decision tree algorithms to make predictions of patients' survival. Using these algorithms for regression problems has been discussed in more detail in Chapter 10. In this chapter, we do not delve into the details, and only compare models' performance by comparing RMSE.

For creating our regression model, we use the `tree()` function of the "tree" package [12].

```
> library(tree)
> DT_reg <- tree(Survival~., data=reg_train)
> summary(DT_reg)

Regression tree:
tree(formula = Survival ~ ., data = reg_train)
Variables actually used in tree construction:
[1] "PRAME"  "CHI3L2" "SAA1"
Number of terminal nodes:  5
Residual mean deviance:  74.79 = 2244 / 30
Distribution of residuals:
   Min. 1st Qu.  Median    Mean 3rd Qu.    Max.
-17.850  -5.692  -1.501   0.000   5.649  18.550
```

Of the five independent variables, only three of them have been used in making the predictions. This holds valuable information provided by the rest of the two independent variables from our predictions. In order to see the effects of the exclusion of these variables on the model's performance, we compare the model's RMSE with the rest of regression models.

```
> predict_DT_reg <- predict(DT_reg, reg_test)
> RMSE_DT <- rmse(predict_DT_reg, reg_test$Survival)
> RMSE_DT
[1] 11.15099
```

RMSE for our decision tree model is higher than the rest of regression models, which is due partly to the exclusion of independent variables. Similar to decision tree classifiers, decision tree regression models can be pruned after being developed to their full potential. This can be done using the "rpart" package, which interested audience is encouraged to apply to prune the model.

Random forest for regression

Random forest regression models showed best performance in predicting neuroblastoma patients' survival among the regression models discussed in this book. We assess its performance using the real-world data set in this chapter.

```
> library(randomForest)
> RF_reg <- randomForest(Survival~., data=reg_train)
> predict_RF_reg <- predict(RF_reg, reg_test)
> RMSE_RF <- rmse(predict_RF_reg, reg_test$Survival)
> RMSE_RF
[1] 8.676893
```

Since random forest decreases the risk of overfitting to training data, its predictions on unseen data are more accurate compared with other algorithms such as decision tree.

K-nearest neighbors for regression

KNN uses feature similarity to predict the value of a new data point based on already existing neighborhoods. The number of neighborhoods (*K*) can be chosen by analysts and then modified or methods such as cross-validation can be used to report the optimum number of neighborhoods. Principles of creating a KNN for regression problems are similar to that of classification problems. We use the `train()` function of the "caret" package for this purpose, and we use cross-validate to find the best K value.

```
> library(caret)
> reg_KNN <- train(Survival~., data=reg_train,
+                  method="knn",
+                  trControl=trainControl("cv", number=5),
+                  preProcess=c("center", "scale"),
+                  tuneLength=30)
There were 50 or more warnings (use warnings() to see the first 50)
```

As was mentioned before, the warning messages are not a cause of worry, and are due to the relation between the number of the variables and the values tried for *K*. We now compare the model's RMSE with previous models.

```
> reg_predict <- predict(reg_KNN, reg_test)
> RMSE_KNN <- rmse(reg_predict, reg_test$Survival)
> RMSE_KNN
[1] 10.50079
```

Our model has better performance compared with linear regression, SVM, and decision trees, which can be attributed to nonparametric features of this algorithm. Furthermore, cross-validation used in training the model reduces the chances of overfitting on the training data.

Neural networks for regression

As mentioned earlier in this chapter and Chapter 13, neural networks are powerful algorithms for making predictions. However, these algorithms work in their full potential in large data sets, which allows them to perform their pattern recognition. We also mentioned that if our observations can be linearly separated, it is better to not use neural networks for training predictive algorithms. Considering these limitations in our data, let us compare the RMSE of a neural network with three nodes in the hidden layer with other regression models developed in this chapter.

```
> library(neuralnet)
> reg_NN <- neuralnet(Survival~., data=reg_train,
+                     hidden=3, act.fct = "logistic",
+                     linear.output = F)
> predict_NN_reg <- predict(reg_NN, reg_test)
> RMSE_NN <- rmse(predict_NN_reg, reg_test$Survival)
> RMSE_NN
[1] 21.33318
```

RMSE of our neural network regression model indicates poorer performance of this model compared with other regression models. Our observations almost follow a linear trend, as was shown with plotting our LR model, which further justifies poor performance of neural networks in making predictions.

In conclusion, in order to choose the best predictive model for our data, whether it is a regression or classification model, there are several parameters to be considered. First and most important is the nature of our data set, including but not limited to the number of the features and observations, as well as the distribution of observations. Considering these factors helps us rule out certain algorithms. The other factor is characteristics and assumptions of the algorithms. Even though some of the assumptions of algorithms are almost never met in real-world data, extreme deviations from these assumptions can dramatically affect the model's performance.

References

[1] M. Kuhn, Caret package, Journal of Statistical Software 28 (5) (2008).

[2] W.N. Venables, B.D. Ripley, Modern Applied Statistics with S, Fourth edition, Springer, New York, 2002.

[3] J. Fox, S. Weisber, An {R} companion to applied regression, Third edition, Sage, Thousand Oaks CA, 2019.

[4] Revelle, W. (2021). Psych: Procedures for Psychological, Psychometric, and Personality Research. Northwestern University, Evanston, Illinois. R package version 2.1.9.

[5] Meyer, D., Dimitriadou, E., Hornik, K., Weingessel, A., Leisch, F., Chang, C. C., et al. (2021). e1071: Misc Functions of the Department of Statistics, Probability Theory Group (Formerly: E1071), TU Wien.

[6] T. Hothorn, K. Hornik, A. Zeileis, Unbiased recursive partitioning: a conditional inference framework, Journal of Computational and Graphical Statistics 15 (3) (2006) 651–674.

[7] Therneau, T., Atkinson, B., Ripley, B. (2019). Rpart: Recursive Partitioning and Regression Trees.

[8] Milborrow, S. (2021). Rpart.plot: Plot 'rpart' Models: An Enhanced Version of 'plot. rpart'.

[9] A. Liaw, M. Wiener, Classification and regression by random Forest, R News 2 (3) (2002) 18–22.

[10] Fritsch, S., Guenther, F., Wright, M. N., Suling, M., Mueller, S. M. (2019). Neuralnet: Training of Neural Networks.

[11] Hamner, B., Frasco, M., LeDell, E. (2018). Metrics: Evaluation Metrics for Machine Learning.

[12] Ripley, B. (2021). Tree: Classification and Regression Trees. R package version 1.0–41.

Index

Note: Page numbers followed by "*f*" and "*t*" refer to figures and tables respectively.

Printed in the United States
by Baker & Taylor Publisher Services